D0032633

THE
HERBAL DETOX
✦✦✦ PLAN ✦✦✦

OTHER HAY HOUSE TITLES
OF RELATED INTEREST

Books

The Allergy Exclusion Diet:
The 28-Day Plan to Solve Your Food Intolerances,
by Jill Carter and Alison Edwards

The Body Knows:
How to Tune In to Your Body and Improve Your Health,
by Caroline Sutherland, Medical Intuitive

Eating in the Light:
Making Your Way to Vegetarianism on Your Spiritual Path,
by Doreen Virtue, Ph.D., and Becky Prelitz, M.F.T., R.D.

Healing with Herbs and Home Remedies A–Z,
by Hanna Kroeger

Shape Your Life: *4 Weeks to a Better Body—and a Better Life,*
by Barbara Harris, Editor-in-Chief, *Shape* ® magazine,
with Angela Hynes

Vegetarian Meals for People-on-the-Go:
101 Quick & Easy Recipes, by Vimala Rodgers

Wheat-Free, Worry-Free:
The Art of Happy, Healthy, Gluten-Free Living, by Danna Korn

Audio Programs

Body Talk: *No-Nonsense, Common-Sense,*
Sixth-Sense Solutions to Create Health and Healing,
by Mona Lisa Schulz, M.D., Ph.D., and Christiane Northrup, M.D.

Eating Wisdom, by Andrew Weil, M.D., with Michael Toms

Your Diet, Your Health, with Christiane Northrup, M.D.

All of the above are available at your local bookstore,
or may be ordered through Hay House, Inc.:

(800) 654-5126 or **(760) 431-7695**
(800) 650-5115 (fax) or **(760) 431-6948 (fax)**
www.hayhouse.com

THE
HERBAL DETOX
✦✦✦ PLAN ✦✦✦

The Revolutionary Way
to Cleanse and Revive Your Body

✦ Xandria Williams ✦

Hay House, Inc.
Carlsbad, California • Sydney, Australia
Canada • Hong Kong • United Kingdom

Copyright © 2003 by Xandria Williams

Published and distributed in the United States by: Hay House, Inc.,
P.O. Box 5100, Carlsbad, CA 92018-5100 • (800) 654-5126 • (800) 650-5115
(fax) • www.hayhouse.com • **Distributed in Australia by:** Hay House
Australia Pty Ltd, P.O. Box 515, Brighton-Le-Sands, NSW 2216 • *phone:*
1800 023 516 • *e-mail:* info@hayhouse.com.au • **Distributed in Canada by:**
Raincoast, 9050 Shaughnessy St., Vancourver, P.C., Canada V6P 6E5

All rights reserved. No part of this book may be reproduced by any
mechanical, photographic, or electronic process, or in the form of a phono-
graphic recording; nor may it be stored in a retrieval system, transmitted,
or otherwise be copied for public or private use—other than for "fair use"
as brief quotations embodied in articles and reviews without prior written
permission of the publisher.

Also published in 2003 by Vermilion, an imprint of Ebury Press,
Random House, 20 Vauxhall Bridge Road, London SW1V 2SA
www.randomhouse.co.uk • ISBN: 0 09 188221 4

LCCN no.: 2002115910

ISBN 1-4019-0101-8

06 05   04   03   4 3 2 1
1st Hay House printing, February 2003

Printed in the United States of America

✦ ✦
Xandria Williams

M.Sc., D.I.C., B.Sc., A.R.C.S., N.D., D.B.M., M.R.N., NLP
*Naturopath, Nutritionist, Herbalist, Homeopath, Reflexologist,
Psychotherapist, NLP Practitioner*

Xandria Williams began her career as a geochemist involved in mineral exploration. She then turned to biochemistry and the study of the human metabolism and nutrition. She qualified as a naturopath, nutritionist, herbalist, and homeopath. Later she studied psychotherapy, voice dialogue, time-line therapy, and became a qualified NLP practitioner; and has explored these and other methods of helping people with emotional, personal, and psychological problems as well as physical health problems.

She has lectured extensively over the past twenty years at many natural therapy colleges and at conferences and seminars; she holds classes and seminars on a range of aspects of physical, mental, and emotional health care. She is currently a lecturer at the Institute of Optimum Nutrition and the College of Naturopathic Medicine, both in London. She has a lucid and easily comprehensible style of lecturing and writing, even when covering complex topics, has written over 350 articles, has frequently been heard on radio and television, and is the author of sixteen books, being published in many different countries and languages.

She has used and applied her understanding of the action and use of herbs extensively in her practice, both in the use of prescribed herbal remedies and the use of herbs in culinary ways. She has often had a hundred or more herbs in her garden and uses them extensively herself. Her knowledge of such natural ways to improve health and well-being have led to this book.

Xandria Williams has evolved her unique and highly effective approach to tackling life's problems, physical and emotional, over more than two decades of writing, research, teaching, and helping patients at her clinics in Sydney and London.

Books

Her books include *Living with Allergies, What's in My Food?*; *Osteoporosis*; *Choosing Health Intentionally*; *Choosing Weight Intentionally*; *The Four Temperaments*; *Beating the Blues*; *You're Not Alone*; *Fatigue, the Secrets of Getting Your Energy Back*; *Overcoming Candida*; *Liver Detox Plan*; *Stress, Recognise and Resolve*; and *Building Stronger Bones*.

Supplements formulated by Xandria and available from Nutri Limited at 0-800-212-742.

Liver Support: the nutrients referred to in the *Liver Detox Plan*.

Adrenomax: the nutrients referred to in *Stress, Recognise and Resolve*.

Xandria is currently in practice in central London and can be contacted for consultations or copies of her books:

28 Lower Sloane Street, London SW1W 8BJ
Phone: 020-7824-8153 • E-mail: xkw@bigfoot.com

✦ ✦
Contents

✦ ✦

Introduction

DETOXING IS IN DANGER of becoming a buzzword, yet it has a profound significance. As the years and decades go by, more and more chemicals are being made, used, and pumped into the environment, the marketplace, and your body. They enter through your body via your food, drink, medications, and anything else you may swallow via the air you breathe, your skin, and anything else you may insert into any orifice — scares over tampons is an obvious example. More and more health problems are occurring that do not constitute a specific disease or illness that a doctor can treat, yet they leave the individual feeling unwell with a range of sometimes vague and sometimes specific symptoms.

Increasingly, people are seeing naturopaths and related natural therapists and saying, in effect, that they feel toxic, and they think they need a good cleanout. This has been abundantly clear in my own practice, particularly since I wrote the *Liver Detox Plan* a few years ago. Clearly, the content of that book hit a chord with a lot of people.

For decades now, we naturopaths have been warning against the dangers of agricultural and food additives, of environmental toxins, and the dangers of physical forces such as microwaves and mobile phones. We have warned of the dangers and toxic effects of medical drugs and the damage that is done to our food supply as a result of the way foods are processed. Some people have heard, but others refuse to hear — either because it is too much bother to change their lifestyle, or because they have a vested interest in the current practices.

For years we warned against the dangers of margarine made by hydrogenating vegetable oils. Gradually, the established medical world is beginning to recognize the dangers posed by the trans fatty acids (altered fats) that form as these margarines and other products containing hydrogenated fats are produced. These

1

dangers include an increased risk of several types of cancer, atherosclerosis, and heart disease.

For years we have warned people against the dangers of overheating fats in food processing, saying that this process and the foods produced in this way greatly increase your risk of developing cancer and a number of other health problems. Such overheated fats occur in nearly all fried foods and particularly in deep-fried foods such as chips, potato chips, or burgers. They also occur in foods, particularly those containing fats, such as meat or baked goods, whose cooking involves high temperatures or the searing of the outer surfaces — foods that have been roasted, barbequed, grilled, or char-grilled.

Now the Food Standards Agency has finally acknowledged that fried, baked, and other foods containing overcooked fats contain acrylamide, a substance that can cause infertility, damage the nervous system, and lead to mutations and cancer — particularly of the breast, uterus, adrenal glands, and scrotum. The potential damage increases exponentially with increases of temperature required to gently glaze onions or to cook a soft omelette. It is acknowledged that there is no safe dose of acrylamide, though European rules allow ten ppb (parts per billion) in foods. However, commonly eaten foods, such as those above, contain from 20 to 400 times as much, and possibly more.

Toxins, and the damage they can do, have long come of age as a major threat to the health of the population. Dealing with them is a two-step process. First, avoid or reduce, wherever possible, what you take in or are exposed to. You will probably be surprised to find out just how much you can do in this regard, provided you are willing to make the effort and the adjustments to your lifestyle. Some adjustments, it is true, will be major, but many of them are minor, yet they offer enormous benefits. Second, become aware of and put into practice, ways and means of both strengthening your body's defense systems and its ability to eliminate toxins.

+++ PART I +++
The Benefits of Detoxing

✦ ✦ ✦

IN THE *LIVER DETOX PLAN*, I discussed the role of the liver, the thousands of reactions it carries out in the maintenance of normal health, and the consequences to you if it becomes damaged or overwhelmed by toxins itself. I also wrote about the huge role it plays in detoxing the rest of your body and what you can do to maximize its effectiveness.

Now I want to look at what you can do with herbs to encourage this Detox process. In the following chapters, you will learn about and, I hope, come to respect, herbs. You will discover how they can improve your digestion, prevent the formation of toxins within your gut, increase the elimination of waste and toxins — and do so several times, not just once a day or less. You will learn about herbs that boost the function of your immune and lymphatic systems and about blood cleansers as they collect and transport toxins to the exit points. You will learn about herbs that help your lungs and kidneys and increase your elimination of toxins via these routes. You will discover that many problems, including skin problems, fluid retention, and obesity, can be caused by toxins; and that herbs can help you deal with them.

I hope you will also come to realize that a huge range of health problems, which you may think of as inherent diseases or disorders, are actually clusters of symptoms that are due to the presence of toxins. You will then understand that these problems can be eliminated by dealing with these toxins, and that the judicious and generous use of herbs can be a powerful tool with which you can achieve this result.

Easier Weight Loss

Have you spent weeks on a strict diet and not lost weight? Have you, in the past, been able to diet relatively successfully but suddenly found that, no matter what you do, the weight simply won't budge? The answer may relate to the level of toxins in your system.

From the moment of birth — in fact, even before that — even in the uterus, you are exposed to toxins. They may be physical or chemical; they may be solids, liquids or gases, but one thing is certain: a large number of them have in common the fact that they are either chemicals or produce chemicals, and that these chemicals are fat-soluble rather than water-soluble. There would be little point in adding water-soluble pesticides to plants; they would get washed off in the first rain that fell. And there is little point in adding water-soluble gleamers to fresh fruit to improve their looks, as they too would soon wash off.

No, most of these toxins, the chemical additives to our foods and to animal feeds, are fat-soluble. In addition, toxins that are water-soluble are quite likely to have been lost from your body in the urine. It is the fat-soluble ones that your body has trouble with. If the liver cannot break them down and if there is no suitable carrier system to eliminate them, many of them are stored. Where are they stored? Initially in your liver, to be dealt with later — but its capacity is limited — and the rest are stored in your body fat, in that unwanted adipose tissue that adds inches to your measurements.

It has been suggested that when your adipose tissues are too toxic, your body is reluctant to break them down. After all, as you lose weight and the fat is released and taken to the various cells to be used for energy, the toxins would also be released and left to wander around your bloodstream. As they traveled they would pass through your brain, heart, and other organs, and have the potential to do all sorts of harm. Certainly I have found over the years that a number of patients report an unexpected and unexplained weight gain at some time in their life. When we explored the details, it has often turned out that it was associated with a sudden increase of toxins.

I recall one man who started gaining weight suddenly after he went on an extensive course of medical treatment. The weight went on with the drugs but stayed on long after he had stopped taking them. All efforts at dieting failed until he went on a Detox Regime. Then, without even trying to cut calories or reduce the amount he ate, he started to lose weight, slowly and steadily and with little effort.

Another patient, a woman of nearly 280 pounds, had a similar experience. She had been through an unpleasant, traumatic, and prolonged divorce. During that time, she had stopped bothering to cook proper meals, and had subsisted mainly on processed and chemical-laden, prepackaged meals. She had eaten sweets, drunk considerable amounts of coffee and alcohol, doubled her cigarette intake, and become a habitual user of sleeping pills and headache tablets. A year or so after the settlement, she finally decided to do something about her weight. She had tried a variety of diets, from crash diets to serious calorie restriction. Nothing had worked. I put her on a Detox Regime where she used many of the ideas discussed here and took supplements that help to tie up or "green bag" (see p.18) the toxins. I also emphasized that she should not consider herself to be on a diet, a suggestion that in itself reduced a lot of her tension, but simply that she was trying to get healthier. In no time, the weight was coming down at the rate of a steady pound or two every week, and both she and her life were getting back into shape.

There is another aid to weight loss involved here. Once you start on a Detox Regime and begin to feel the benefits of it, you will want to continue. It may seem hard at first to give up some of the things you love, such as the toxin-laden, calorie-laden, high-fat foods, but once you feel the benefit, things change. So many patients have said this to me.

I recall one women who just loved cheese. She ate out in restaurants frequently, both in her work and socially. No matter what she ate or how much, the cheese board at the end of the meal was always a temptation she could not resist. On went the calories. After a month of forced abstinence, as she went on a Detox Regime, she lost all interest in cheese. Her first mouthful, at the end of the month, she said was an eye-opener. As she described it: "It tasted and felt like a lump of greasy lard, and after all the work I had done and after feeling so good, so 'clean' and so supple and fresh, I didn't want to put it in me anymore."

Another patient said he had come to prefer the light, crunchy texture of fruits and vegetables and the refreshing feeling of them, compared to more solid and heavy foods.

What does all this mean for your weight? It means that once you are firmly on a Detox Regime, you will find yourself preferring the beneficial foods, naturally favoring those that are also helping you lose weight, rather than the high-calorie ones that encourage weight gain.

You will find out how to set up your own Detox Regime below in Part XI and feel the weight fall away.

Increase Your Energy

Do you ever feel too tired to cook? Are you too fatigued to take care of yourself properly? Does it seem like too much effort to bring about the changes in your life that you know, if you are honest with yourself, could make a big difference to you? Is there nothing actually wrong with you, yet you find your get-up-and-go has got up and went?

Many patients come in and tell me that there is nothing really wrong with them, they just don't feel right. They feel sluggish; and they have lost their motivation, their concentration, and their enthusiasm for life.

Valerie was like that. She suffered from sinus headaches and said they were worse in the mornings when she had eaten a big meal late the previous evening. Clearly her digestive system was sluggish. Yet by the end of the day, she was often too tired to cook so she bought a package meal from the supermarket, got take-out, or made do with snacks and nibbles. Her best evening meals were when she ate out with friends, but that usually meant a late meal with a heavy intake of alcohol, often in a smoky atmosphere.

It was a vicious cycle, and one that she finally resolved to break. Together we worked out an eating plan for her and incorporated in it lots of the herbs you will read about later on. After a few days with a furry tongue and some noticeable changes to her digestive system, she reported feeling a lot more clear-headed, her sinuses unclogged, and she felt a lot more energetic — energetic enough, as she put it, to shop for and prepare a meal for herself when she got home so that she had the energy to break the insidious cycle.

However, it is not always plain sailing. One woman came to me saying that she knew she was eating a lot of rubbish; she knew she worked in a polluted environment. Worse still, her business life involved entertaining at lunchtime, and her social life was built around eating out with friends. She did not want to give up any of this. I assured her there was no need to. You can eat perfectly well, even when you eat out; it is simply a matter of making sensible choices when the menu is presented to you and drinking a lot more water and somewhat less alcohol.

For her, we built a lot of fresh vegetables, fruits, and salads into her restaurant choices. She'd start with a salad, choose a light fish dish with plenty of vegetables, and, if the meal was prolonged, have some fruit for dessert. She switched to peppermint tea after meals to help her digestion, took some of the other herbs described below, and was still able to enjoy her social life. Another tip worked well for her. At my suggestion she always asked for a second wine glass and a bottle of mineral water. She found that half the fun of drinking was the physical action of holding the elegant wine glass and sipping *some* type of drink. This way she was able to increase her water consumption, an important part of a Detox Regime, and reduce her intake of alcohol without anyone else noticing or commenting and without in any way spoiling her enjoyment of the occasions. When she discovered how much more energy she had as a result of doing this, she vowed she would stick with the Regime for life.

Improve Your Brain Power

Mental fogginess, poor memory, poor concentration, lack of mental alertness, headaches, lack of motivation, apathy. Are these some of the problems that bother you? The great thing about cleaning out your system is that it is not only your body but your brain that is "cleansed." Increased mental alertness almost always comes with it.

Many of the toxins that we surround ourselves with are brain toxins. They fog up your thinking. You would be well advised to get rid of the silver amalgams in your teeth. Mercury makes up more than 50 percent of these amalgams, and mercury toxicity is a problem. The aluminium in most commercial and chemical antacids is another brain toxin. Swap to the methods described below for improving your digestive system, and you will no longer need these aluminium-laden products and your brain function will improve.

Many other toxins can fog up your brain. It is a lot easier to think clearly when your sinuses are clear and your nose is not blocked. It is difficult to concentrate and be mentally alert when your digestive system is sluggish, when you feel nauseated, or when your abdomen is so bloated you look pregnant. Herbs can help solve all these problems for you.

An essential part of a Detox Regime is water. Depending on the nature of your diet, you should aim to drink between one and two quarts of water a day. If you eat mainly fresh fruits and vegetables, including a fresh salad daily, then your fluid intake can be slightly less than if you eat a diet made up of foods that contain less water. As long as your intake is adequate, this too will help improve your memory and your brain power.

I recall a patient who had been a successful self-employed accountant but had been forced to retire early because he was becoming forgetful and finding that his brain, as he said, had gone fuzzy — so much so that he had started making mistakes and felt he was letting his clients down. Once he started on a Detox Regime and particularly once he got into a routine of drinking a pint of water three times a day an hour or so before each meal, all this changed, and he started to restore his practice to the point where it was interesting but still gave him the time to pursue his other interests.

Get Rid of Those Headaches

Do you suffer from headaches? Do you wake up with them, or do they develop during the day? Many toxins can lead to headaches. A sluggish and toxic liver can cause them, too. Blocked sinuses and a congested nasal passage can lead to headaches. There is no need to suffer in this way. If headaches or migraines are a part of your problem, then one of the groups of toxins that may be contributing to the problem could be allergens. It could well be worth having a test for food allergies. If you have them, once they are identified and you avoid them and do this in combination with going on your own Detox Regime, the headaches and migraines could become a thing of the past.

Make Your Skin Glow

Would you like to have better skin? Would you like to lose blemishes, reduce gray shadows, and look radiant? It is almost impossible to have toxins in your body and not have them show up on your skin. They can manifest in many different ways. You may simply have pale, dull, and lifeless skin, instead of a glowing complexion. You may have the gray shadows and/or bags under your eyes associated with a sluggish liver or kidneys. Perhaps whiteheads and blackheads are part of the problem. Or it could be worse. You could have pimples and boils or cysts, you could have bad acne.

Do you regularly use additional makeup to hide the blemishes? Do you hate to be seen before you have your makeup on? Do you wear a beard to cover the blemishes? Perhaps the problem involves the rest of your body. Do you get pimples all over your back and therefore hate to uncover in the summer?

Once you have started on your Detox Regime the benefits will be obvious. The blemishes will go, the color will return, and your skin will take on a whole new glow. So many patients, coming in for an entirely different reason but following my suggestions as to lifestyle and diet, have reported that friends are telling them they *look* different, that their skin glows, and they look healthy.

No Need for Colds

More patients than I can count have come to me saying that they suffer from frequent colds, when in fact the diagnosis is quite different. What they take to be repeated colds are often frequent bouts of sinusitis or periods when they produce large amounts of mucus. This may be the result of exposure to substances or the consumption of foods to which they are allergic. Or it may be that the body's way of eliminating toxins is by producing the mucus and other symptoms that they think of as having a cold.

One patient found that allergic reactions to cheese and wine were causing his frequent colds and his permanently blocked nose. He gave them up for the most part. However, he had an excellent wine cellar, and when the urge to take out a bottle became too much, he found that if he also drank infusions of some of the expectorant herbs discussed here, his reaction was far less severe than he had been used to.

Another women had recently, along with her husband, fulfilled a lifetime dream and bought a pub. All went well in the summer when the doors and windows were open most of the time. The problems started in the winter. What she thought was a nearly constant cold — brought on, she presumed, by the heavy work-load and long hours — was in fact her body's response to the smoky atmosphere. By using the expectorant herbs in combination with blood cleansers, she found that she could eliminate all the symptoms, and she also felt a lot more energetic and capable of both doing the job and enjoying her new life.

Protect Your Heart and Your Arteries

Most people take their heart and arteries for granted — that is, until they get older and their cholesterol is found to be too high or friends start having heart attacks. Cleaning up your act can also benefit your heart.

Take a minute to consider what happens when you eat fats. When these fats are first absorbed from your diet, they enter your bloodstream in the form of large, low-density, globby balls called chylomicrons. These chylomicrons are transported through your bloodstream and deliver some of their fat load to cells (that want it for energy), or they take it to your liver. In your liver, there is a general reshuffling, and these fats emerge incorporated in smaller and slightly more dense lipoproteins called Very Low Density Lipoproteins or VLDLs. These VLDLs continue to deliver some of this fat and eventually become compounds called Low Density Lipoproteins or LDLs.

Other changes, such as the nature of the protein, occur in the liver, which is critically important to your body's proper manage-ment of the fat you eat. These LDLs deliver their residual choles-terol to the many different parts of your body that do need it and so become the heavier HDLs or High Density Lipoproteins. These eventually return, gather up the "spent" cholesterol, and return with it to your liver.

If your liver fails to fulfill all these functions correctly, then a number of problems can result that can have a negative effect on your blood fats, your arteries, and your heart. If your liver is overwhelmed by toxins, it has reduced capacity to handle your blood fats properly, so a detoxed liver will undoubtedly help your heart and your arteries.

There are other considerations. Toxins that you take in from your lungs or digestive tract, including those inhaled from cigarette smoke, travel through your bloodstream. As they travel, they cause damage to your artery walls leading to atheromas, blocked arteries, and heart attacks. Provided your liver is detoxed and ready, it can deal with these toxins sooner rather than later, and so reduce the harm they can do. If you both reduce your intake of toxins *and* improve the capacity of your liver to remove the rest from your bloodstream as fast as possible, you will be able to protect your artery walls and the health of your heart.

Improve Your Sex Life

It is difficult to have a happy sex life if you suffer from vaginitis, frequent episodes of candidiasis (thrush), or herpes. By eliminating toxins from your system, you can reduce your symptoms and improve the situation. You may do this by improving the function of your liver, digestive system, or kidneys. You can further improve the situation by using immune-boosting herbs, anti-fungals, and other herbs specific to your particular problem. As a result, there need be no more days when you feel uncomfortable and wonder about embarrassing odors. There won't be any more nights when you have to say no when you would really prefer to say yes.

. . . and More

If some of these benefits to a Detox Regime come as a surprise, be warned, because there are more. When you eliminate toxins from your life style as far as you possibly can, and when you use the suggestions and herbs described here to improve your health, tone up your whole system and Detox, you may become even healthier than you had expected.

✦✦✦   ✦✦✦

+++ PART II +++

What Toxins Are
and What They Can Do

✦ Chapter 1 ✦

What This Book Is All About

So LET'S GET STARTED. Do you feel tired and run down? Are you groggy in the mornings, sluggish throughout the day, and tired before bedtime? Is your skin spotty, pasty, and looking old before its time? Do your sinuses bother you, or do you just seem to get frequent colds? Does your digestion let you down, or does your system cause you gassy embarrassments? Do you suffer from headaches or migraines? Would you like to be lighter and slimmer, more alert and energetic, and look and feel younger? Do you have any health problems you would like to get rid of?

If you answer yes to any of these questions, then you could find answers in the following pages.

Are you in perfect health, physically, mentally, and emotionally where health is measured not as the absence of symptoms but as a state of perfect and exuberant well-being? Does your body function perfectly, never causing you a moment's worry or concern? Do you laugh at the thought of needing a doctor? Is your skin clear and glowing, your hair glossy and shiny? Are your nails strong? Are you free from all aches and pains? Do you sleep easily and well, waking refreshed and ready for each new day? Do you eat a good diet that includes lots of fresh fruits and vegetables and drink at least two pints of water a day? Do you have three easy bowel motions a day? Have you ever thought of herbs as helping to solve any of your health problems?

If you answer no to any of these questions, you could, again, find the answers in the following pages.

It may surprise you to know that all the problems mentioned and many others can be caused by the toxins that surround you and that enter your body on a daily basis.

Shortly we will be learning a lot more about toxins. You may feel that you know what they are and what you should be doing to avoid them, but you may also be in for some surprises. You might find that many of the things you take for granted in your life and consider to be harmless can actually turn out to be very harmful indeed. The mere fact that they are permitted in our food supply, in the home, and in the atmosphere does not mean that they are harmless. There are permitted food colors and additives, permitted medical drugs, permitted social and industrial practices, and permitted pollutants. This does not mean that they are completely safe. Thousands of people die annually from the toxic side effects of medical drugs. Thousands more suffer illness resulting from their use. More thousands are thought to be suffering from the effects of mobile phone, electro-magnetic radiation, radioactivity, food additives, and more.

The toxins that surround us all include chemical, physical, and biological toxins. Many of them are obvious, others come hidden — undetected by sight, smell, taste, or touch. Many are not even recognized. It is all too easy to take current habits and behavior patterns as normal and assume they are safe. I frequently hear comments such as: "Other people do it, so it must be all right" or: "It can't be bad for you or it wouldn't be allowed." Not true, of course, as people are starting to realize. Other toxins come lauded for their benefits. It is easy to praise the chemicals that stop molds forming on food, the drugs that kill individual pathogens, the sprays that keep your home clean and the food processing that allows you to spend less and less time in the kitchen, yet ignore the harmful consequences of these substances and practices that are hidden, at least temporarily.

You *can* avoid some of these toxins. You can do a great deal, for instance, to avoid many that are ingested or used in the home. You can do less to avoid others, such as the electromagnetic radiations that pervade the ether and the industrial and social pollutants dispersed throughout the air you breathe, although even here, there are some things you can do.

Even one day in my practice throws up a number of examples of people suffering ill health as a result of the toxins to which they are exposed. In a year, there are many, many more examples, some of them particularly memorable.

Jennifer, in her late 40s, came to me with a variety of vague mental and neurological symptoms; her doctor had told her they were probably due either to multiple sclerosis or a mild stroke. It turned out that she was reacting to the toxic mercury released from the amalgams in her mouth. The subsequent removal of this toxin solved her problems.

Louise had a history of fifteen years of bad health. When we identified and removed her allergens (foods that were toxic to her) from her diet, she felt so well that she furiously bemoaned the stupidity of the past fifteen years of needless suffering.

Steven suffered from eczema and bronchial and sinus problems — all of which disappeared when he stuck to organically grown and produced foods and used herbs that helped clear his lungs.

Anita had for years used copious makeup to cover the teenage acne that had extended into her thirties. When she modified her diet, increased her fluid intake, and took the recommended herbs, all her symptoms went away.

Deirdre had suddenly gained 42 pounds over a period of a few months and couldn't lose it no matter what diet she tried. After going on the herbal cleanse, she was able to lose weight just by eating carefully.

Martin had a high-powered city job and was permanently tired and irritable. Using a colon cleansing program that involved diet and herbs, his energy came back with a rush, as did his efficiency and mental clarity.

Since you are reading this book, it is likely that you have some health problem that has bothered you for a while. Perhaps it is one that keeps recurring. Perhaps it is one that the doctors have tried to treat, but without success. Perhaps you have problems that do not constitute a named disease and you have been told they are all in your mind, that you are suffering from stress or that you need a good holiday. Perhaps you think you are imagining things, or becoming a hypochondriac. You may have tried a number of solutions but with little result.

Or perhaps you are interested in staying well and in using herbs to help you maintain good health. Perhaps you are aware of at least some of the damage toxins can do and want to learn as much as you can about them and how to both avoid them and minimize the harm they can do.

How do you deal with your own situation? First, it is important to learn all you can, so we will start off by discussing the basics. Then it will be time for you to take action. The solution is three-fold.

- First, you must avoid or reduce your exposure to toxins wherever possible. Advice on how to do this is found below.
- Second, you must build your health so that you reduce your vulnerability to the toxins that you cannot avoid. You can do this by using specific herbs outlined in Part IV.
- Third, you must get rid of the toxins you have already accumulated. If you are currently not in perfect health, we have to assume that you start with a load of toxins already on board and already doing you harm. As a result, you will need to follow a specific Detox Regime to get you off to a good start. I will help you design one to suit your unique needs.

There are a number of Regimes you can follow. They range from fasting on water or juices, through mono diets such as eating nothing but brown rice or fruit, to various specific Detox Regimes such as the one detailed in my *Liver Detox Plan,* or the herbal-based Regime detailed later on that uses both diet and herbs.

You could choose a mono diet, but a word of warning is important here. It is important that your Detox Regime does not cause unnecessary side effects along the way. Think of spring cleaning. If you go at it like a demented lunatic, flinging out all the rubbish, intent only on having neat and tidy cupboards with no unwanted old possessions stuffed away in the corners and no dirt anywhere, you may finish the day with wonderfully neat cupboards, but the living areas of your rooms will be a shambles of piled rubbish and dirt. These you will then disperse through the rest of your house or apartment, too tired to clear them away before you collapse exhausted into bed. The next day you will still have a large part of the work to do to clear up the new mess you have created.

If, on the other hand, you clear out one cupboard at a time, carefully putting the rubbish or dirt into green bags, one for paper to recycle, one for plastic, one for composting, and so forth, you will achieve several aims. First, you will gradually achieve, step by step, a wonderfully tidy house. Second, you will do it without creating any further mess that can be trampled throughout the system, causing new havoc. Third, you will have done it in an environmentally friendly way and, finally, you will have done it by creating new habits that you can continue to follow.

It is the same when it comes to spring cleaning your body. You do not want to stir up all the rubbish and cause more pollution. Phase I involves mobilizing the toxins stored around your body. However, you do not want to mobilize toxins from their stored fat deposits, for instance, and leave them to wander around in your bloodstream, coursing through your brain and other organs and causing a range of side effects. You do not want to create headaches, a furry tongue, bad breath, nausea, or any other new symptoms, or even aggravate these if they are already present. It is better to detox in a controlled manner and wrap up (green-bag) the rubbish as it is mobilized so it doesn't cause even more symptoms. This is Phase II.

What does this mean? For one thing, it means that a simple water or fruit fast may not be your best option. You may release the toxins from their stored depots, but they may circulate and do harm. It means that you should use a program that encourages safe and rapid elimination from your body, as well as from individual tissues. Designing a personal herbal Detox Regime will give you the best overall results. You can choose to incorporate the herbs best suited to your health problems.

In addition to eliminating toxins, a Detox Regime should include methods of boosting your immune system and reducing the harm that can be done to you by viruses, bacteria, and other pathogens. You will also have to avoid or deal with the known toxins that have entered the food chain, causing such things as salmonella, BSE, and a range of other problems. You can incorporate immunity-boosting herbs into your Regime.

The next section of the book will be all about herbs. Herbs can play many and profound roles in helping you to clean out your body, improve your energy, and keep you healthy. Some of these herbs are medicinal and hard to come by, particularly as government legislation is making it difficult to acquire or market herbs, although you can still get many of them via the Internet.

More of this later (see p.75). You will also find that a surprising number of common culinary herbs, or those that are readily available as teas or simple remedies, have a lot to offer. They can be purchased easily and are readily incorporated into your lifestyle. If you are even more interested in this approach, you will find that many of the herbs mentioned either grow wild or are available from garden centers, and you can grow your own. I will explain how herbs are prepared and in what forms they can be taken. You will also find plenty of recipes incorporating many of the individual herbs discussed.

Then it will be time for you to think about some of the many problems that may exist throughout your body's systems. You may find you have some health problem that you thought was predetermined, inherited, or due to some infection or a degenerative disease but that can actually be solved by cleaning up your act and eliminating certain toxins. It is both sad and exciting to find how easy it is to "clean out" some health problems. It's sad because years of needless suffering may have passed, but it's exciting because excellent health can be restored relatively easily. You will find advice on herbs specific to those health problems.

Have you ever considered how your body gets rid of the toxins you take in or produce? Few people have. Yet it is often the blocking of this elimination process, perhaps through your lungs or through your skin, that leads to unexpected health problems. Mucus of itself is not bad, it is part of the mechanism by which your lungs expel toxins. A temperature of itself is not bad, it is the way your immune system is able to activate its defenses faster and for infection-fighting enzymes to work more efficiently. If the problem is recognized for what it is — the presence or formation of unwanted toxins — and if the elimination process can be encouraged rather than suppressed until your body is clear, you can then get better faster and prevent the development of further problems.

There are many methods and routes that can be used to eliminate toxins. One of the main organs that deals with toxins is your liver, and in *Liver Detox Plan,* I dealt with this in detail. But your liver is not the only organ involved. Other organs and systems are also involved in elimination and detoxification, and they include the various organs of your digestive system, your kidneys and urinary system, your skin, your lungs and the rest of your respiratory system, your lymphatic and immune systems, and your bloodstream. You will be reading and learning about all these and how to help every system in your body to function better.

The next part of the book will involve incorporating everything you have learned, and developing your own Detox Regime. You will find a detailed four-week plan with strict dietary advice to follow, but with room for you to choose the herbs that suit your own needs. You may be surprised by how many changes can be brought about by simple herbs and the ease with which it can all be done without dangerous side effects.

You will also discover just what efforts you have to make to get the desired results. Some people think the effort well worth it, others decide they can't be bothered.

I know one man who gives up all alcohol for the first three months of the year. It's his New Year's resolution and commitment. Within days of starting this regime, his energy doubles, his mood improves, and things that only days earlier had made him fly off the handle are now dealt with calmly and constructively. By Easter, however, the regime has begun to pall, he celebrates with champagne, and gradually returns to the old problems, at least until next Christmas.

Just as some considerable changes may be required to get all the results you want, you may be surprised to see just how easy it is to achieve some positive benefits. You may find that by making some simple lifestyle modifications, you can transform a lingering malaise into exuberant health and abundant energy. Or you may decide that now is the time for a major change and rethink the way you are leading your life.

A patient in Australia was told by her fiancé shortly before their marriage that he had decided to enter the church and, what's more, to go to a seminary in New York. Devastated, she upped her intake of alcohol, junk foods, sugar, chocolate, tea, coffee, and the number of cigarettes she smoked. Depressed and miserable, knowing you cannot fight God, she sought comfort where she could until, thoroughly run down, she came to see me. I made many of the usual suggestions, including the one that she should make the changes at her own speed.

To my surprise and pleasure, when she returned two weeks later, she had completely transformed her life. Out had gone the old habits, completely, cold turkey. She had emptied her kitchen cupboards. Sugar, white rice or flour, processed foods, coffee, tea, chocolate, alcohol, or cigarettes — all were given to friends. In went organic foods. She raided the health food stores, bought books on healthy living, became a near vegetarian, started growing sprouts and pot herbs in her apartment, and salad greens on her balcony. She had benefited not only her health by direct action, but emotionally by having a new and interesting project to pursue.

Finally, you will find information about where you can find herbs. I hope you will be pleasantly surprised by how easy it is, and find plenty of ways to help yourself by using them.

The Herbal Detox Regime in this book is a plan to help you clean out your system. It will help you to eliminate stored toxins in your body. It will teach you new habits such that you minimize your exposure to toxins, and maximize your ability to deal with the ones you can't avoid; it will teach you to do this harmlessly and safely. Ultimately it will teach you how to improve your health, looks, and energy, and to maintain the good results you achieve on a lifelong basis.

The Regime is based on a sensible lifestyle, good eating, and the constructive and beneficial use of herbs on a daily basis. And if all this makes you think: *Boring, boring, I'll have to give up all the things I enjoy and have no fun anymore,* you may also be in for a few surprises. It is just as easy to eat out and socialize in a healthy way as in a toxic way, unless of course you prefer to eat junk foods and maintain bad habits. It is just as easy to keep your house the way you want it by healthy means as by the use of a range of toxic products. There may be a few sacrifices you have to make, but think also of the rewards. Ultimately this choice is yours. As one patient said to me: "It costs a bit to get and keep healthy, but gosh, being sick costs a great deal more."

✦✦✦   ✦✦✦

✦ CHAPTER 2 ✦

The Naturopathic Perspective

IT IS APPROPRIATE, FOR A MOMENT, to divert to a discussion of homeopathy, for reasons that will quickly become clear. In classical homeopathy, as first developed by Hahnemann, there were very few toxins either in the environment or in our foods compared to the vast number to which we are exposed today. In most instances, an illness had a symptom pattern that was specific to that illness and the way it manifested in that person. Similarly, a remedy had a specific symptom pattern. It was then a case of matching the remedy, known as the similimum, to the patient's symptom pattern and prescribing accordingly.

Today the situation is different. A pattern of symptoms is generally the result of a combination of factors. There may indeed be the specific illness itself. But almost certainly the symptoms are overrided by and combined with the symptoms resulting from a wide range of other factors including food and environmental toxins, vaccinations, altered combinations of microorganisms, and other pathogens. If any medical treatment has been tried, for this or for any other problem, there will also be the overlay of the side effects of the drugs used. Since much of the aim of allopathic (drug) medicine is to suppress or eliminate symptoms, rather than to effect a complete and fundamental cure as understood by naturopathy and homeopathy, the picture will be further distorted.

As a result of this, a situation has developed where frequently there is no single homoeopathic remedy, taken from the mineral, plant, or animal world, that is likely to exactly match a complex overlaying and interweaving of symptoms such as this. Thus, in modern homotoxicologically based homeopathy, it is rare to use the similimum or single remedy as was done decades ago. Instead, a two-fold approach is frequently taken. First, a much greater focus is placed on recognizing which of several, increasingly severe, levels of toxicity the person has progressed to. Steps are then taken to bring them back, level by level, to less deeply ingrained levels of disease. This is done by using a carefully selected combination of homeopathic and other remedies in combination with detoxification procedures, rather than by using a single similimum. The process is further assisted by modifying the diet and lifestyle.

There are several reasons why I have chosen to discuss and emphasize this here.

- It is important to further emphasize the importance and power of toxins in the development of most health problems or groups of symptoms that occur in the 21st century.
- It is important that you recognize these toxins and avoid them in any future health-care program in order to maintain whatever benefits you achieve.
- It is of vital importance that a Detox Regime is an integral and essential part of any effort to improve your health and well-being.

If homeopathy has had to change its emphasis, in just two hundred years, then the changes that have taken place in our environment and our health in that time are profound. This same situation is recognized in other branches of the natural therapies, though perhaps in a less structured way and without a specific name having been coined.

In herbal medicine, for example, great emphasis is placed on the alterative herbs. These were once known as "blood cleansers." They are now recognized as ones that have the general effect of restoring normal function within the body and producing a general increase in energy and health, a clear recognition of the importance of detoxifying the system. The description itself indicates the importance of cleansing or detoxing in the restoration of optimum health.

In nutritional-based therapies, there is an emphasis on organic and unprocessed foods as well as on those that contain and provide the maximum levels of nutrients, followed by supplements that help to support detoxification processes as well as provide additional tools for the positive function of whatever part of you is suffering.

In naturopathy, emphasis is placed on fasting, fruit or juice regimes, or other cleansing diets as part of the general healing process.

These are all manifestations of the recognition of the need for detoxification as well as for therapy.

✦✦✦   ✦✦✦

+ Chapter 3 +
A Toxic World

WE LIVE IN A HIGHLY POLLUTED WORLD. In some instances, this is so obvious that it is almost commonplace. We know there is pollution from industry, urban life, traffic, and many other sources — we can smell it and see it. We know of and read about pollutants spoiling our rivers and lakes and killing our wildlife. We know there are unwanted chemical additives in our food and dangers from biological sources like BSE and salmonella. People are so concerned about the purity of their water supply that millions of dollars are spent annually on bottled, purified, and filtered water. People are sufficiently concerned about the agricultural pesticides added to fruits and vegetables, grains and meats, and about the chemicals that are added during food processing that the market for organically grown and produced food is growing and threatens to outstrip supply.

Other toxins are less obvious. You may not realize that the lemon-scented, country-fresh spray you are exhorted to use to remove the odors in your kitchen contains a veritable cocktail of chemicals that do you more harm than good. The oven spray could be harming the caverns of your lungs. Bleach may clean and whiten your linen and working surfaces, but it generally contains oxidizing agents that generate free radicals and harm many of the tissues throughout your body. These free radicals can be sufficiently powerful that they cause cancer and a range of degenerative diseases. The cosmetics that improve your looks use toxic chemical dyes to create the colors and hues; the powders and creams that sweeten and hide your natural body odor can seem harmless, yet contain talc (a silicate rock), harmful minerals, oils (that leach vitamins from your body), aluminium, and other toxic chemicals. And before you walk into the shower or sink into that hot bath and lie back to relax, think about all the chlorine, a powerful oxidizing agent, that is being given off while the water is running. You would be well advised to run the bath while you are not in the room, and open the window to let much of it out. For the same reason, when you flush the toilet, put the lid down first.

There are thousands of food additives, from those that are used during the farming and growing of the foods to those used in the many stages of transport, processing, and storage through to the ultimate product. Read labels. Most have toxic chemicals, permitted in small amounts but not guaranteed to be safe, just *generally thought* to be *acceptable*. We like food to look good. Most people prefer their dried apricots to *look* like apricots and be a nice bright orange, ignoring the fact that sulphur compounds are added to the fruits to preserve the color, compounds that can change into toxic acids in the moist interior of your digestive system. Try adding fresh strawberries to plain yogurt yourself. Do they produce the stark pink color of the purchased product? No, of course not. Think about the colored gums that are given to children as sweets and tremble at the thought of all the petro-chemical dyes that have gone into them.

There is another problem. Since the chemicals are there in small amounts and many of them, other than the obvious dyes, are colorless, they cannot generally be seen, and it is all too easy to ignore the possibility of their presence. Imagine what would happen if all the added chemicals that you eat in a year, estimated to be well over two pounds, were collected together and put into bottles on a shelf. I'm sure, if asked to, you would refuse to eat them and recoil in horror at the very idea.

Some toxins are idiosyncratic: safe for other people but harmful for you. There may be foods that you cannot eat without your body reacting adversely and developing a number of unwanted symptoms. Most people may eat these foods as part of a good diet and suffer no harm, but for you they may cause trouble. These foods are sometimes called allergens; they are sometimes referred to as foods to which you are sensitive.

There is a school of thought that says certain foods are good for you and others should be eliminated from your diet on the basis of your blood type. These blood type markers, so the hypothesis goes, combine with certain foods, causing the blood to agglutinate and possibly lead to other problems. If your blood type is O, you would do best on a Stone Age diet of flesh foods and most (but not all) fruits and vegetables. If your blood type is A, you should avoid meat and rely on chicken, many types of fish, and most (but not all) fruits and vegetables, your selection of these being different from type O blood people. If your blood is type B, you can, with more ease than the other types, include dairy products in your diet. And if your blood type is AB, you have the slightly more difficult task of, in general, avoiding the foods that should be avoided by both type A and type B, although you can handle dairy products better than the type As. In my clinical experience, this has helped some patients considerably, although others report little change in their symptoms.

The most common social drugs are chocolate, tea, coffee, alcohol, and nicotine, and they contain many toxins; some are more toxic than others. Some do more harm to some people than to others, but they all do harm nonetheless. Recreational drugs are even more damaging. All medical drugs have some toxic side effects, sometimes relatively mild, at other times severe, up to and including being life-threatening. The severe side effects can be sufficient to create new illness and health problems in the process of trying to eliminate the old ones.

Physical forces such as electromagnetic fields are harmful. They include problems inside the house such as around your television set, computer screen, electrical blankets, the batteries, and other electrical appliances. Other problems are created outside the house and include the electromagnetic field from transformers, power cables, and mobile phone relay stations. Radioactivity is toxic.

Many biological forms are toxic, ranging from small single-celled bacteria to more complex worms and other parasites.

Then there are the waste products and toxins you produce yourself. In the normal course of the day, even when you are healthy, you produce a range of waste products that have to be eliminated. The protein you eat contains nitrogen that is converted into ammonia or urea and has to be eliminated as waste products, usually via your kidneys; otherwise, it goes to your brain, where it is potentially lethal, as in cases of liver failure. The cholesterol you eat, although having great value, eventually has to be eliminated, this time via your liver, gallbladder, digestive tract, and colon. The steroid hormones you make must eventually be eliminated in the same way. The carbon dioxide you produce, as a result of producing energy from food, has to be eliminated by your lungs.

The toxins that you make within your body include the toxins created in your colon if you are constipated. These can be created by simple putrefactive chemical reactions or by pathogenic organisms that should not be there but that thrive in conditions that are the result of poor stomach acid production, of constipation, or improper digestion.

It is hard to define toxins in a simple statement as to their nature since they are so many and so diverse. Rather we might take the broad approach and base the definition on what they do. A toxin is anything, substance or force, that is harmful to your body, your health, your looks, your energy, to your physical, mental or emotional well-being. Toxins can be chemical, physical, or biological; they can also be mental. If you increase your level of worry, resentment, or anger, you can generate chemicals that are toxic and have to be dealt with by your detox system. If that is already overloaded, this may reduce your capacity to deal with other physical toxins.

This is not a book about toxins. It is a book about detoxing your system and about the herbs you can use to do so. To find lists and descriptions of environmental toxins and the specific harm they each can do, you need to explore further, as there is not sufficient room here to cover all those details. However, through suggestions made here as to how to clean up your act, change your life, and reduce your exposure, you will get many indications of toxins, and mention will be made of many as we progress.

Toxins enter your body in many different ways. Some arrive with food or drink and are swallowed. Others are coughed up from your lungs and swallowed, or ingested after you have taken in breaths of polluted air through your mouth without the filtering benefit provided by your nose.

Others are inhaled. These may be gases or very small particles. They may enter your lungs by invitation. Cigarettes are an obvious example. Others come in uninvited. You have to breathe. But you do have some control. You can choose when you breathe in or out, and you could elect to breathe out (or hold your breath) when that large truck drives past spewing noxious fumes.

Substances with which you come into contact, or that you apply to your skin, can be absorbed through your tissues. Where else do all those creams and lotions you rub on to your body go? Talcum powder, high in aluminium compounds, applied to your armpits is thought to be absorbed and has reportedly been found in the liver. Whether this is by skin absorption or inhalation hardly matters. That lipstick you keep replacing doesn't all go on the glass or cup, much of it is swallowed. Oils, dirt, grease, paints, marker pens — all these can sit on your skin, and some can be absorbed before you wash them off.

Other routes include injections or entry via other orifices. For instance, that perfumed douche you use may well contain substances that are not so pleasant, some of which you may absorb.

By now you will be getting some idea of the toxins in your world and how they can enter your body. They can be the cause of almost any health problem you care to name. At best, they can leave you feeling slightly under par, not ill but not well either. At worst, they can be responsible for major illnesses, including cancer, and even death. Their effects may come about immediately, in the short to medium-term or in the very long-term. It may be clear what toxin caused what problem or it may not. Usually it is the latter. You will probably never know just what it is that is making you feel unwell. Be wise, though, and recognize that if you ignore the problem of toxins, you are blocking a major route back to good health.

That is a brief indication of some of the major types of toxins with which your system has to deal. It is now time to consider what happens next, for toxins can cause problems in many ways.

- They can cause local problems as you absorb them. They can create problems in your mouth or digestive system. Your lungs can be damaged by the irritant effect of inhaled toxins. Your skin may be irritated by what you put on it. They may not even be harmful when consumed, but be converted into harmful compounds on the way in.
- Toxins can also cause harm as you excrete them, problems to your urinary system or colon.
- And if you don't eliminate them but choose to store them instead, they can almost certainly do you harm for as long as they remain. Let's explore these ideas.

Trouble on the Way In

Some toxins can do immediate damage as you take them in. They may cause problems in your mouth, set your teeth on edge, or give you heartburn. Others are actually changed into toxins as you take them in.

The nitrates used on meats are a case in point. Mentioned briefly already, these nitrates of themselves are not toxic. The problem comes when you swallow the treated meat. The nitrate combines with the amino acids of the meat protein in the presence of the acid in your stomach to make compounds called nitrosamines. It is these nitrosamines that are toxic and are thought to be carcinogenic.

What do the nitrates do? When added to the meat you buy, they do three things. They kill bacteria, keep the meat looking bright red and fresh, and add to the general "meaty" flavor, particularly of bacon and similar products. I have seen ground beef, allowed to grow old and green with age, then dunked in a nitrate solution and then coming up looking bright red and fresh. It would have fooled any keen-eyed person into thinking he or she was buying truly fresh meat.

I have heard butchers defend its use on the grounds that it prevents the infection of the meat with pathogenic bacteria. This is true, but there other ways of doing that, ways that are safer for the consumer. But these other ways do not keep the meat looking bright red, nor do they add to the flavor, so they are not the preservatives of choice from the butchers' standpoint.

Some of the compounds you inhale when you either smoke a cigarette or inhale second hand are not toxic of themselves. But because they are not water-soluble, they would be carried with difficulty by your blood. As a response to this, once consumed they are hydroxylated and then carried to your liver. This may make them easier to transport, but it also produces compounds that are more toxic than the original.

Trouble on the Way Out

Many toxins can do harm even as you eliminate them. For instance, carrying a load of toxins through your digestive system can cause problems to your colon. This will be particularly so if you are constipated. Since you probably eat three meals a day, it would be reasonable to assume that you should have three bowel movements a day. If you do not, then some food waste is sitting there for longer than normal before being expelled. If you don't even go once a day, then the problem is a lot worse. While this waste food, with its content of toxins, is sitting, and probably fermenting, in your colon, a number of things can happen. The toxic compounds themselves may, while they are waiting, be absorbed through your colon wall and into your bloodstream.

In addition, as a result of the fermentations and other chemical reactions that can occur during that time, new toxins can be generated, and they too can be absorbed into your bloodstream. In fact, one test for toxins in the bowel, called the urinary indican test, utilizes this fact. By doing a simple analysis on a urine sample, you can determine the presence or absence of a toxic substance that indicates a high toxic load in your colon and the absorption of these toxins into your bloodstream and their transport to your kidneys.

Many toxins lead to the production of mucus experienced in your bronchial tubes and nasal passages. These substances can be universal toxins, inhaled particles, or aggravating chemicals. They can also be foods that are safe for most people but toxic to some with a tendency to allergies. Dairy products are particularly prone to leading to the production of mucus, but grains and other foods can also do so in some individuals. If the toxins in your system show up as an excessive production of catarrh, you may be prone to repeated bouts of bronchitis, or experience what you think of as frequent colds when all that is really wrong is an overload of these allergenic toxins. This catarrh, as it sits there waiting for you to either blow your nose, or sniff and swallow, is an excellent breeding ground for pathogenic bacteria that in turn can generate more toxins for you to absorb, either through your lungs or by swallowing into your digestive tract.

When toxins are eliminated through the skin, you may surely notice the result. Toxin-laden pimples, whiteheads, or blackheads are unsightly and the bane of many people's lives. Especially as their most common positions are the face and the back.

There are even more complex ways in which toxins can cause harm on the way out.

Marion had been told by her doctors that she had multiple sclerosis. She had also worked out for herself that she was, as she put it, allergic to vitamin C. Every time she ate fruit, sweet peppers, tomatoes, lettuce leaves, any other food with a high content of this vitamin, or took a vitamin C supplement, all her symptoms got markedly worse. Since it is unlikely that anyone is actually allergic to a vital nutrient such as vitamin C, we decided to explore the situation further. It turned out that her multiple sclerosis symptoms were actually due to lead toxicity, the symptoms of which can mimic those of this disease. It then seemed likely that each time she consumed a significant amount of vitamin C, her body mobilized some of this stored and toxic metal. This lead was then carried around her body, causing an aggrava-tion of her symptoms before finally being eliminated in the urine. Her solution was a treatment with chelating agents that bound the lead; immediately it was mobilized, in such a way that it did minimum harm on the way out.

Later on, when we discuss what the liver does, you will find there are two steps to detoxification and elimination. Phase I involves mobilizing the toxins from wherever in your body they are stored. Phase II involves conjugating or combining these compounds with other substances so that they are not free to do further damage as they are eliminated. Again, it is a bit like the process of spring cleaning when first you clean out the cupboards and put the waste into green bags so it does not fly around the rest of the house. These rubbish-laden green bags can then be carried out of the house and left outside for garbage collection. Later you will learn about the important role your liver and a number of nutrients and herbs play in "green bagging" these toxins so they do no harm on the way out.

Trouble When They Stay

Perhaps these comments, particularly those about the harm toxins can do in the process of being eliminated from your body, have made you think twice about going through a detoxification process.

Don't hold back. It is important to stress that in general, toxins do far more harm when stored, particularly if you take a long-term view. For instance, toxins stored in the liver will gradually damage your liver, with harmful consequences for nearly every aspect of your health (see the *Liver Detox Plan*).

Not all toxins can be dealt with or stored by your liver. They have to go elsewhere. Most of them are soluble in fat rather than in water, and these are therefore easily stored in your adipose tissue, those unwanted fat stores you are usually trying to eliminate or minimize. The result is toxic-laden, fatty tissue. This will cause some, but minimal, damage while your weight remains constant and the toxins remain safely stored. They will cause some problems, as your tissues are never static. All the time some of your fatty tissues are being broken down (as your cells demand fat for energy) and then replaced (as you consume a high-calorie meal with excess fat to store).

The situation changes the moment you decide to lose weight, as we noted briefly at the start. Then these toxins will cause more problems. First, they will make it more difficult for you to lose weight as your body becomes reluctant to release the toxins back into your system. Second, as you do lose the unwanted weight and the adipose tissues are broken down, the stored toxins will be released. They will circulate throughout your body and brain on their way out, causing a variety of symptoms both physical and mental. The presence of toxins may even encourage weight gain as your body tries to create places to store the toxins.

I recall a patient, Robert, who had suddenly started to gain weight after he'd gone abroad to work in a country where the availability of fresh food was limited. He attributed the problem to the high-calorie foods he had eaten there but was surprised when he returned home, improved his diet, and still could not lose weight, no matter how little he ate. After a Detox Regime, the diet started to work, his weight went down, and his health improved.

Some of these stored fat-soluble toxins can be held in the fat-protein complexes that circulate in your bloodstream. The fat-protein complexes are the lipoproteins we discussed earlier when considering the benefits to your heart of eliminating toxins. You will recall that there are several different types, including the Very Low Density Lipoproteins (VLDLs), the Low Density Lipoprotiens (LDLs), and the High Density Lipoproteins (HDLs). The important ones from our point of view are the LDLs. These are the lipoproteins that are present in increased amounts when your blood cholesterol level is raised, and many researchers think it is the toxins that these LDLs carry that damage the artery walls and lead to atheromas, atherosclerosis, and heart disease rather than the cholesterol itself.

You probably already recognize that stored toxins can affect your skin, and indeed your skin is one of your organs of elimination. As toxins are secreted, they can lead to whiteheads, blackheads and pimples, they can lead to a gray color and pasty skin tone. You cannot have fresh glowing skin when your system is toxic.

Stored toxins can affect your brain; the way you think; and the way you feel, emotionally and mentally. They can lead to fuzzy thinking, poor concentration, reduced memory, and lack of initiative and motivation. They can make you feel cross and irritable and can even cause mental diseases.

Stored toxins can interfere with your immune system, damage your bones (where they can also be stored) and joints, and in fact cause harm to almost every part of you.

There may be some problems that arise during a Detox Regime; however, these can generally be minimized. Stored toxins can cause harm for years, for the rest of your life, setting up a variety of present and future health problems. A properly managed Detox Regime can be simple, fun, and almost instantly rewarding. This is particularly true if you understand what you are doing and know how to do it properly.

The Healing Crisis

You may have heard some naturopaths talk about a healing crisis. They may consider it a necessary part of a Detox Regime. This concept deserves some consideration. In the 19th century and the early part of the 20th, there were relatively few toxins around; they were also relatively harmless. As they were mobilized from the body's tissues, transported through the bloodstream, and eliminated, they could do little harm. You might have gotten a headache, a furry tongue, a slight feeling of nausea, or a mild temperature. Then these, the components of the healing crisis, would have passed, and exuberant health would have resulted.

Nowadays the story is different. Because the toxins are so much more potent, because there are so many of them, and because they can interact to produce a veritable cocktail of toxins with unpredictable results, more care must be taken. You may still get a headache when you stop drinking coffee and other caffeinated drinks — that is, a caffeine withdrawal headache — but there is nothing to be done for it except take a "hair of the dog" and drink some more coffee. However, this only prolongs the agony and the temptation should be resisted. In any case, no painkillers will help. All you can do is put up with it for a day or so and then promise not to become addicted again and so have to repeat the performance.

In general, however, it is no longer acceptable, nor is it a good idea, to simply fast, put up with a healing crisis, and wait for better health. If, when you go through any Detox Regime, the ones suggested here or any other, you find that you are developing new symptoms, it is time to seek professional advice. The toxins of our world are too dangerous to be allowed to run rampant throughout your body.

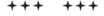

✦ CHAPTER 4 ✦

Reduce Your Exposure

Cleaning Up What's Around You

THE FIRST STEP TOWARD DETOXIFICATION is to reduce the toxin load
to which you are exposed. We will accept that there are some
toxins about which you can do little, at least on a daily basis.
However, it is estimated that a huge proportion, probably the
majority, of the toxins to which you are exposed come from sources
which you can control — both by what you buy, eat, and drink,
and by how you live your life.

As we go through the list, you may find yourself saying: "But
that is just a tiny amount, surely it can't matter." Remember that
pennies are very small coins, but enough of them can make you
a millionaire.

So, let's go through a typical day. I make no claim that this list
is absolutely comprehensive. Since I use so few toxins myself, I
am often surprised, when visiting the homes of other people, to
find what they are willing to use.

We'll Start in the Bathroom

Cleaning Do you need that foaming soap (usually detergent
based)? There are some lovely natural* [footnotes are at the end
of Part II] soaps on the market. You may like bubble baths, but
herbal oils give a wonderful fragrance to a bath and are better for
your skin. Include pine or rosemary oil for stimulation. Use
chamomile or lavender oil in your evening bath for a relaxing sleep.
Moisturizers Consider the various lotions and potions you use.
Many of them could be replaced by more natural products.
Remember it is your intention and hope that they will be absorbed
into your body, so make sure they are toxin-free. Even the
absolutely basic baby oils and hand and body creams we all grew

up with can cause problems. Most of them are based on petro-leum derivatives. Instead, use ones derived from vegetable oils or lanolin. Petroleum oils, if absorbed into your body (which is what you expect to happen), are not broken down or metabolized. Instead, they pass though unchanged. Because they are oils, they can pick up some of the fat-soluble vitamins in your body and take them out with them, thus depleting your stores of these valuable nutrients.

Aerosol sprays Get rid of aerosol sprays for a start. There is nothing — no hairspray, hair treatment, perfume, deodorant, or anything else — that cannot be bought with a pump spray instead of an aerosol. Even if you don't mind the harm they do to the atmosphere, you don't want to breathe in the toxins from an aerosol.

Deodorants Avoid deodorants that contain aluminium or come as aerosols. There are plenty of roll-on creams. Try using simple aloe gel; it results in healthy skin that does its job properly.

Cosmetics Read the labels and consider what you could be doing to your body. When considering cosmetics, there is a difference between those that are not tested on animals and those that are natural. The former are not necessarily free from toxic chemicals,* which is one of the reasons they need to be tested. The latter, from natural sources such as lanolin, vegetable oils, and essential plant oils, do not need such testing. Natural cosmetics and toiletries include those produced by Wala and Weleda in the UK.

Toothpaste Check your toothpaste. What's in it? Do you really want to put that in your mouth? Certainly you spit most of it out, but not all. There are many excellent ones available in health-food stores based on herbs: herbs that help to deter candida and other molds; herbs to kill various bacteria; and herbs such as pepper-mint or fennel for the flavor rather than using chemical flavors.

Alternatively, you could use the following combination: aloe vera gel first, then a couple of drops each of propolis tincture and grape-fruit seed extract; add them to the brush sequentially as you clean. The former is excellent to help heal bleeding gums, and the latter two are antifungal and antibacterial. The sodium form of vitamin C, as powder, is helpful. Be careful not to use the acid form, ascorbic acid, as it will harm your teeth, and the calcium form is also best avoided. But sodium ascorbate is excellent; put a small pile on your toothbrush and brush away. You are mashing vitamin C into your gums, just where you want it to both help heal bleeding gums and boost your immune system's fighting capacity

Drugs Check your medicine cabinet. Do you really need half the things that are in it? Aspirin? Why not solve the problem that causes those headaches? Antacids? There are much better and more appropriate solutions to heartburn (see p.106). Antiseptic creams? Apply sodium ascorbate powder as a paste. Vapor rubs and balsams? There are many excellent herbal alternatives available from your health-food store. A few brief sessions with a naturopath could provide much healthier solutions to almost all the quick-fix drug remedies in your medicine chest.

Now the Kitchen

Aerosol sprays Again, get rid of all those aerosol sprays. Simple pump actions will achieve the same results without all the extra chemicals polluting your environment, to say nothing for what they are doing to the ozone layer.

Cleaners You will probably find enough toxins in the cleaning cupboards and under the sink to cause untold damage. You may feel that you need them to keep the house hygienically clean. However, you can now buy a wide range of natural cleaning products including detergents for the sink and the dishwasher, and laundry soaps for woolens, general washing and washing machines, and bleaches and toilet cleaners. Which would you rather have: a detergent made of plant-based surfactants, milk whey, salt, citric acid, herbal extracts including chamomile and marigold and a preservative; or a chemical detergent that declines to tell you what's in it and advises you to avoid prolonged contact between it and your skin?

It may be true that the natural detergents do not cut the grease quite as well as their chemical counterparts, but think about what you are doing. That strong chemical detergent residue may attack the grease on your dirty dinner plate, but when left on your plate after washing (and they are very hard to rinse off entirely) it becomes incorporated into your next meal. It can then "cut" or damage the lining of your digestive tract, to say nothing of the harm it can do if absorbed into your body.** At the very least, use the natural ones most of the time and resort to stronger cleaners only when they are absolutely needed.

It may also be true that the natural products cost more than their chemical counterparts, but there is nothing so cheap as a cheap product, as we will discover when we consider different foods. It is also true that you are dealing with your health. This is often accorded little value until you lose it, then it becomes priceless. If you think keeping healthy is costly, wait until you discover the true cost of restoring your health once it is damaged. **Others** Check your other kitchen cupboards, and keep in mind that some authorities have suggested that as much as 30 percent of your toxins come from your own kitchen. Consider what you could do without, or replace with a less toxic product. Are the perceived benefits really worth it?

The Next Steps in Your Day

If you travel to work, walk or run where you can. Go by side roads rather than the main ones where all the gas fumes are. If you need to walk where vehicles are belching clouds of exhaust, then hold your breath as the largest trucks go by, and let at least some of the pollutants dissipate before you open your lungs again. Avoid inhaling as you walk past someone who is smoking. Sit in the back of the bus rather than riding near the open door. Such steps may seem small, but remember those pennies.

At work, use the stairs rather than elevators or escalators. Keeping fit is part of the detoxification process. If you have the option, open the windows rather than using air-conditioning. Avoid sitting in front of electrical units such as air-conditioners and heaters. Choose light bulbs rather than fluorescent tubes, but if you have little choice, at least try not to sit directly under the fluorescent lights. If using a computer screen is an intermittent part of your job, angle it so that you are not facing it directly, then turn to it as and when you need to. Use ballpoint pens rather than felt-tips that give off the odor of the ink they contain.

Be wary of smells. It is not enough to say that they are not too bad and you can put up with them. When you detect a smell, it means that molecules of that substance are entering your nasal cavity and attaching to the receptors there. Remember, they can be doing you harm even if you don't detect them. But don't resort to yet another aerosol-delivered chemical spray promising freshness as it covers up the warning odors. Buy fresh flowers instead.

Hopefully you are beginning to get ideas as to other ways you can reduce the type and amount of toxins to which you are currently exposed. If you are at home during the day or going shopping, the same types of considerations apply.

Many jobs have their own particular toxic risks. You will have to research these for yourself and do what you can to avoid them and minimize the damage. Remember, it's worth it. It's those pennies again.

Back home for the evening, there is more to think about. You're about to cook your meal. In what? If you have aluminium saucepans or cooking utensils, they should be replaced with less toxic ones. Choose good-quality stainless steel or Pyrex instead. Be wary of those nonstick pans. They are lined with chemicals that eventually wear off. Where do they go? You've guessed it. At least some of it enters the food and then your body.

Do you really have to use a microwave oven? There is always the chance that they are giving off dangerous radiations if they are faulty. If you use gas appliances or gas heating, have these units checked regularly to make sure no unwanted gases are entering your atmosphere. Keep windows open where possible, but choose the ones where the least amount of pollution can get in. Don't slouch *in front of* the television. If you must slouch, at least do so to one side and as far from it as possible. Be wary of the back of the television, too; the rays can pass through walls and can also do harm.

If you use a mobile phone, be careful. Hold it as far from your ear as possible, keep up-to-date with whatever safety devices are recommended, and talk briefly. Most lengthy discussions can wait until you can use a land line.

Watch What You're Doing

Why not make a conscious decision to have an awareness day. Choose a typical day, but one when you will have the time to pay attention to what you are doing. Go through that day focusing on everything you do with toxins and pollution in mind. Each time you put something on your skin, into your mouth, or into your environment, ask yourself what it consists of, what chemicals it contains, how you could be taking them in, and what they could be doing to you. If you are not sure that their actions are totally beneficial, consider what better alternatives you could use.

Take that same analytical assessment with you each time you go shopping as well. So many toxins, so many unnecessary and harmful chemicals, have crept into our everyday life that even if you think you are doing everything right, you may find that there are still several simple improvements you could be making. Keep up-to-date. Ingredients can change, even on a product you thought was safe.

Mrs. J was elderly, arthritic, and had poor eyesight. She was also gluten sensitive and had to avoid wheat, barley, oats, and rye. At my suggestion, she had sought the help of an assistant in the supermarket to establish just which products were safe for her to eat, then she stuck to those. Some months later, she came back in complaining of her old symptoms. Joint research by the two of us established that wheat flour had recently been added to the cartons of soup that had previously been safe for her to eat.

These and similar changes could make a significant improvement to your health, now and in the future. The future is the problem. As with all preventive medicine, the trouble is that you won't ever know what you might have prevented; you have to take that on trust. However, a quick comparison with other people who have been much less careful will often provide a guide.

All this may sound rather daunting, but it will not be something you think about all the time, only while you are making the initial changes. After that, much of it becomes a matter of simple routine. If there are toxins you decide you simply cannot or don't want to remove, then so be it. Make the changes you are willing to make, and accept the hazards from those that you cannot or won't.

Cleaning Up What Goes Inside You

Now it's time to think about what you consume. Start with your water supply. At best, it contains chlorine, which is a strong oxidizing agent, harmful to bacteria, it is true, but also harmful to you. Boiling will remove much of this, but then it is in the atmosphere and you may inhale it. However, there are many other toxins in most tap water. If you want to remove them, a filter will do a small amount of good. However, the best results are obtained by either passing the water through a reverse osmosis membrane or by distilling it. If you decide not to do either of these, then buy spring water. You are looking for a pure and natural spring water; it may or may not be rich in minerals. This pure water should be used for drinking, both hot and cold, and for all cooking purposes — from making soups and sauces to boiling potatoes, rice, and pasta and steaming vegetables.

Now look along your food shelves. Read all the labels. All those foods with food coloring listed among the ingredients should go. It is true some food coloring are harmless, even vitamins have them. Our taste buds have been so assaulted by the chemical flavors and enhancers of modern processed foods that frequently they have become numb. It may take a little time, but if you switch to natural foods, you will soon come to recognize and enjoy their subtle flavors again.

Ideally, all the foods you cook with should be recognizable as something that came out of the ground on its own. Buy whole tomatoes, not a red puree of unknown origin; fresh fruit, not a whipped-up chemical mousse; real meat and vegetables, not an over-processed packet of powder claiming to be chicken soup. In this way, you can be sure you are not eating overly processed food.

Do you really need to buy packets, tins, or cartons of soup with their various added ingredients? It takes but a moment to pop a lot of cleaned vegetables into a pot, cook them, and, if you wish, liquidize them with some cream and fresh herbs. Buying processed cereals is often an expensive business. You may find you are paying a lot for the packaging and the air it contains. The same amount of money could buy you porridge oats, delicious raw when soaked in milk or fruit juice, and eaten with chopped fresh fruits. Why buy white bread with its addition of bleaching agents, yeast extenders, stabilizers, mold inhibitors, and preservatives when you could buy a simple wholemeal loaf with just yeast and sugar to start the process. Look at your fruit yogurt and other desserts; would the simple addition of apricots to plain yogurt create that strong yellow color? Of course not; some chemical dye is clearly needed to achieve this look. Do you really want to consume it?

Wherever possible, buy organically grown food. It is exciting to find that so many people are now doing this that demand is now beginning to outstrip supply. Hopefully this will increase the enthusiasm of farmers who want to convert, and the willingness of the government to increase the funds it will provide in subsidies during the changeover period.

Personally I dislike the stores that scatter their organic goods among the processed foods. I do not want to have to look for organic beans among the beans section, organic rice among the rice section, and organic nuts among the nut section. I can only presume that the rationale for this is that I might be seduced into buying the non-organic ones if organics are not available. I won't. In general, I will only buy organic produce, to go with what I grow for myself, and I'm not going to waste time in this needless search. I head for the stores that group all their organic produce in one spot.

Expense may be an issue, but take a look in your regular shopping basket. What you spend on organic vegetables you could save by omitting that tub of (expensive) prepared coleslaw. What you spend on organic fruit you could save by leaving out that expensive chocolate mousse or that fat-laden bag of potato crisps. Your kitchen shelves are almost bound to contain a number of relatively expensive products that have little or no food value and are laden with unwanted toxins. And remember, cheap foods are cheap, health is priceless.

Consider growing at least some of your own food. Even if you live in an apartment in a city, you can still grow sprouts. An empty jam jar with muslin and an elastic band is all you need to sprout a range of seeds. Mustard and cress are the classics; alfalfa sprouts are highly nutritious. You can sprout any viable seeds from sunflower to lentils, from soy to chickpeas. Try soaking chickpeas in water for 24 hours, and keep them wet for the next couple of days with occasional soakings until tiny shoots begin to appear. You can now eat them raw instead of using the gas needed to cook them for several hours. They are highly nutritious, being inherently "fresh." They are tasty on their own; or, add a few drops of olive oil and dust them with paprika or powdered herbs.

Even in an apartment you can grow fresh herbs. Instead of the usual pot plants, grow a small sage bush, fresh basil, or a window box of chives. I once visited friends in a tiny apartment in a large German city. They had two ten-foot square rooms, and on the windowsills of each they had erected a series of window boxes in which they grew lettuce, tiny carrots, radishes, and (up either side of the windows) tomatoes and beans. The moment a plant is picked, its nutritional status declines. By growing your own, you can eat them straight from the ground.

If you have a garden, no matter how small, you might be surprised by just how much you could produce. You may argue that you live in a polluted city and that this is no place to grow vegetables, but think of the alternatives — of all the chemicals added to the commercially grown alternatives. At least when you grow your own you are in control.

You can now drink organically as well. My kitchen library includes an organic wine catalog of over 50 pages of organically grown wines from over 14 countries. You can buy organic beer, cider, mead, and spirits including brandy, grappa, vodka, and gin. Even your tonic or ginger ale can now be organic. When you taste the difference compared to the ones you have been drinking, you will recognize the harm the latter have been doing.

What about eating out? Eating in restaurants and with friends is an integral part of the social fabric for many people. I am not suggesting that you become a recluse, eating nothing but your own organic produce. However, you can make good and bad choices. In restaurants, select simple starters such as avocado, melon, or a salad rather that something in a white flour pastry shell lashed up with a colored and flavored creamy sauce. Choose good-quality plain food rather than overcooked and highly processed meals. This is not a book about nutrition, but it is certainly true that not only are most desserts an unhealthy mound of fat and sugar, but they are also usually laden with a lot of other unwanted and often toxic additives.

Even when eating with friends, you can make wise choices. You do not need to fill up on those fat-rich and chemically flavored, appetizers. You can dodge the worst of the sauces and desserts and you can set a good example by what you provide in your own home.

✦✦✦   ✦✦✦

✦ CHAPTER 5 ✦

Be Responsible for Yourself

IF YOU ARE TRYING TO DETERMINE what is safe and what is not, there is generally little point in relying on untrained or unqualified people, people with vested interests, or copying what others do and how they look and behave. Other people are fallible, other people have their own sets of benefits, and other people are frequently less healthy than they look. This is the time for you to do your own studying and to make your own decisions. As I've already said, many of my patients say such things as "Other people consume, use or are exposed to these things and they seem to be all right," or "If it wasn't safe it wouldn't be allowed," or "Everybody else does so why can't I?'

At the end of the day, if toxins can cause problems, if you are exposed to them and if you do not minimize this exposure and the damage that they can cause, it is you who will suffer, not someone else. It will not be the people who tried to assure you that everything was fine, safe, and acceptable. Have you ever heard of a doctor being prosecuted for prescribing a medical drug with known side effects? Have you ever heard of a politician who has been prosecuted for allowing a "permitted" food additive with known side effects into the marketplace? It is hard enough trying to prosecute the companies that market such products as cigarette, asbestos, or silicon breast implants — most of them avoid responsibility. Even when such cases are successful, it is still you, the consumer or the person exposed, who suffers the worst harm.

It's a bit like walking blithely across a pedestrian crossing and assuming that the approaching car will stop. If it doesn't, it may be in the wrong, and the driver may be penalized, but it is you who will be lying hurt on the road; it is you who will suffer.

What, you might wonder, is the government doing to let us consume substances that are toxic or be exposed to compounds if they are dangerous? Actually, I suspect that most readers will recognize that the government of the day is a poor watchdog over our health. You only have to think of many of the food scares that have occurred over recent decades to recognize this. The government is just a group of people like you and me. Few politicians have any detailed knowledge of food chemistry and toxicology. They rely for expert advice on the technical committees and advisory panels. And who tries to get on to these committees and panels? That's right — the people from the food industry, those people whose products are being reviewed, or researchers whose grants are funded by the food industry that they are trying to protect.

Perhaps you think the food technologists know what they are doing and would not add harmful substances to their products. Not so. I was dismayed to find, some years ago, that their three-year-degree course included exactly zero hours of nutrition or health care. They are simply taught how to make the best product as judged by its shelf life, public appeal, and profit margin. Any other considerations focus on the ease with which it can be passed through the equipment — packaged, stored, and presented.

Footnote

* Some explanation is needed regarding the words *natural* and *chemical* as used in this book.

Natural applies to substances found naturally in plants, animals, or the human body. Not all natural substances are safe, and you can almost certainly think of a number of natural poisons ranging from the nitrogenous alkaloids in potato and tomato leaves, through toxic mushrooms to various animal products. However, by and large, natural substances are either harmless or more easily detoxified in the body than the thousands of man-made chemicals produced by our current technology.

Chemical is used in this context to mean man-made chemicals that do not occur naturally. It is true that every substance is made of chemicals from air and water through all the biological kingdoms and including all material objects. It is unfortunate that common usage gives this term both meanings, but here the former meaning is used, as is common practice in this context.

** It is important to realize that there is a difference between substances that enter your digestive tract and those that enter your body fully.

Think of your digestive tract as a continuous tube that runs through your body from mouth to anus. You could, for instance, swallow a small glass ball on a string and have it pass straight through you and out the other end without ever having to cross any barriers and with the tail of the string still protruding from your mouth. Substances that pass through this tube can damage the tube itself but, unless they are absorbed further, do not become an integral part of your body.

Once substances cross the walls of your digestive system and enter your bloodstream, they are truly inside you, truly part of you and free to circulate to all parts of your body. The same is true of substances that enter your body via the lungs or through your skin or that are injected directly into either your muscles or your bloodstream.

As a corollary to this, substances that you eliminate in your stool have probably never been truly inside your body, only within your digestive tract. The exception to this is the range of chemicals and bile that are secreted from your liver and gallbladder, or enzymes and other substances that have been secreted in your digestive juices.

Substances you excrete in your urine have inevitably come from your bloodstream and have been truly inside and an integral part of your body.

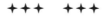

PART III

Detoxification Using Herbs

✦ CHAPTER 6 ✦

Eliminating Toxins

YOU MAY BE READING THIS BOOK for purely preventive reasons, wishing to avoid damage to yourself before any harm can be done, or reading it to help someone else. However, it is probable that you have been leading what I would call a fairly polluted lifestyle, that you have been exposed to a wide range of toxins, and you have been consuming many as well. You may think of it yourself as a toxic lifestyle. You may feel you have, somehow, overdosed on or been exposed to toxins, and that that is why you are feeling less than 100 percent healthy. I hope you might have started to put at least some of the above ideas into practice, and that you are keen to reduce your intake of and exposure to toxins.

It is also important to try to minimize the damage done by those toxins to which you are unavoidably exposed, to excrete them or their derivatives as fast as possible, and to mobilize and eliminate those you are already carrying. It is important to Detoxify.

Before you start a Detox Regime, there are a few important things to consider. When you decide to to spring-clean, you know that during the process there will be a measure of chaos, certainly a mess. There will be piles of rubbish and dust, on the floor or in the bin. Your normal routines will be altered, and in some respects, life may be a bit more difficult for a few days (or however long it takes). What do you do when this happens? You almost certainly don't say: "Gosh, this is making a mess, it is making the place *more* untidy, not less so. I'd better stop and stuff everything back the way it was." Nor do you say. "This is causing new chaos [creating new symptoms] it must be the wrong thing to do." And nor do you say: "This is increasing my activity level [temperature] that must be bad. All this activity can't be good for me. Perhaps I had better leave things as they are and make sure I stay less active."

Most people understand this easily. They recognize that, even with an ever-ready pile of green bags, there will have to be some temporary increases in disorder; there will be some piles of things around the rooms as you sort and tidy. The dustbin will be more full than usual. However, the end point is in sight, you know what to expect, and you tell yourself it will be worth it in the end.

Similar things happen with your body. There is a distinction between unwanted symptoms caused by a badly designed Detox Regime and the healthy symptoms involved in the process of restoring a sick body to optimum health. If you are ill and apply naturopathic, nutritional, herbal, or homeopathic treatment programs you may find that some of them cause a reversal of your old symptoms, usually from the most recent back up to the earliest and usually the mildest. This is a healthy progression. The aim should be to drive the old process out backwards.

Detoxification inevitably leads to the removal of toxins from the body, which may lead to symptoms within your body. The aim should be to keep these symptoms to a minimum, as already discussed when we considered the healing crisis. However, it is also unwise to suppress symptoms. And there is a difference. Many of the symptoms you may experience during a detoxification program are actually those of the body attempting to detoxify and heal itself. If you are unsure of what is happening in your case, you may need to get expert advice.

Modern medicine is generally aimed at suppressing symptoms, including those that are actually signs of the body's own attempt to heal itself. Drugs to block diarrhea, for instance, can reduce the elimination of whatever toxins, chemical, or biological agents, have caused the diarrhea. An increase in body temperature is helpful in dealing with many health problems. Fever should be encouraged, not blocked, by some chemical drug with its own toxic side effects. This is because many of your body's defensive mechanisms function best at a temperature several degrees above normal. In fact, the various reactions that are involved when your immune system is at its most efficient occur ten times more rapidly at 39.5°C (103.1°F) than at the normal body temperature of 36.9°C (98.4°F). The forcible reduction of temperature, by drugs, reduces the body's ability to heal itself and eliminate harmful agents or toxins.

There are several routes to getting rid of your toxins:

- A lot of material is eliminated via your digestive tract in your stool. This includes the nondigestible parts of the food you have eaten, such as the (beneficial) fiber in vegetables, fruit, beans, and whole grains. This fiber also carries with it the old and dead bacteria that have been part of the normal ecology of your digestive tract but are past their use-by date. In addition, it carries the intestinal toxins that have been absorbed onto this fiber (one of the many benefits of a high-fiber diet). These toxins may have come from your diet or they may have been collected up by your liver and passed from there via your gallbladder into your digestive tract. We will discover shortly what this means in relation to the behavior of your digestive tract, how it can be protected from this high load of toxins, and how this route can be improved to increase your detoxification.
- The second important elimination route is via your kidneys, in your urine. Reducing your intake of toxins will take some of the stress off your kidneys. We will also be discussing what you can do to improve your kidneys' function in general and their ability to help in your detoxification program.
- Some toxins are eliminated via your lungs. This is often brought about by an increased production of mucus. We will find ways of maximizing this benefit and then reducing the production of further and unwanted mucus.
- The fourth route is via your skin. This is often the one that troubles people most as it can be unsightly. It means that if you have a number of unwanted skin problems, the solution may well be to decrease your toxic load and to increase the activity of your other routes of elimination so that they do the majority of the work.

Before systemic toxins can be eliminated, they have to be mobilized and transported. Your liver plays a vital role in this as we shall see.

While all this is going on, your immune system has been hard at work fighting all invaders; your lymphatic system has been busy collecting up the toxins that have seeped into your tissues and taking them back into your bloodstream; and your bloodstream itself is carrying all these toxins to their predetermined exit route.

In Part IV, we will discuss your body's systems and these defense mechanisms and eliminatory routes in more detail, what they do for your toxins and what the toxins do to them. We will also be discussing the very important role your liver plays in the Detox process and, of course, how herbs can help at all stages along the way.

We will also be looking at a wide variety of health problems that could be caused by toxins and what you can achieve as a result of the proposed Detox Regime.

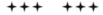

✦ CHAPTER 7 ✦
Herbs — How They Can Help

THERE ARE MANY WAYS OF IMPROVING your detox capacity. To assist in the steps outlined above, the actions of a wide range of nutrients and supplements can be enlisted. In addition, herbs can provide many benefits. You can choose herbs, from a vast range, to suit your own needs.

If you are new to herbal medicine, do not be fooled into wondering how some of these plants that you have probably seen many times in gardens, or in packets on supermarket shelves, can actually have significant medical benefits. These delicate little plants (and some of them not so delicate) contain a wide range of complex compounds. Most of these compounds are important to the plant but may be of little benefit to you. However, many of them also have significant pharmacological properties. Many of these compounds have been chemically extracted by the large drug and chemical companies and have become the basis of modern medicines. They have usually been isolated and modified, which serves not only to alter their action but to allow the products to be patented.

When considering herbs, the first step is to be clear as to what we mean by the term. Strictly speaking, an herb is a "plant whose stem is not woody or persistent." However, this description could include many plants that are not normally thought of as herbs and have no place either in the kitchen or in medicine — many of the common garden and meadow flowers for instance and a lot of weeds. It also excludes many plants that are used in herbal medicine. Trees such as the hawthorn, elder, and elm offer significant health benefits, and their parts are generally included under the term "herbal remedies." In practice the term "herb" is usually applied to any plant that adds flavor to cooking, pleasant aromas to perfumes, or offers a specific health benefit. The term "herbal remedies" covers all natural remedies made from plants or parts of plants of any type, other than foods, of course.

We should also consider the meaning or definition of the term "spice." Many people think of spices and curry in the same breath and think of spices as making foods "hot." In fact, the only spice that makes food "hot" in that sense is chili. All the other spices, such as cumin, coriander, fenugreek, turmeric, and cardamom, simply add flavor. They are all herbs, but with these herbs it is usually the seeds of the plant that are used. They are used more in Indian and Oriental cooking than in Western foods, and so have earned the term "spices." However, you will find that many of these herbs also have medicinal uses and they are in no way "hot."

I used the words "natural remedies" above to apply to herbal remedies. I also pointed out that many of our modern medical drugs come, at least initially, from plants, or parts of plants, but that they have been so processed and extracted that they are no longer considered to be herbs, although their origin was herbal. Consider for instance the foxglove. During past centuries, foxglove, *Digitalis purpurea*, was used to treat heart problems. Then chemists isolated specific active ingredients from it called cardiac glycosides such as digitoxigenin. These glycosides increase the power and action of a failing heart. When extracted from the plant and then synthesized in the laboratory, they lead to medical drugs such a digitalis, digitoxin, digoxin, or similarly named heart medications. Although these medicines were initially derived from a herb, they are no longer considered to be herbal medicines. I recall an elderly herbalist telling me many years ago that when using the herbal extract of foxglove, if you had given too much, you had some early warning signs from other compounds within the plant and could reduce the dose. These early warning signs, he told me, were not produced when the chemically isolated compounds alone were used and thus their use is more risky. In fact, herbalists now prefer to use lily of the valley, which also contains cardiac glycosides but is safer in its action than foxglove.

Let's go back to our discussion of herbs. We have said that the term "herbal remedies" covers all natural remedies made from plants or parts of plants of any type. What do we mean by "parts of plants"? Parts of the plant can include the roots, rhizomes, stem, leaves, fruits, flowers, and seeds. In larger plants, it can include the bark and parts of the bark. All these different parts of the plants have medicinal applications. Some preparations are made from the whole herb, others from the specific part required. The differing parts of the plant can have differing actions. Dandelion, for instance, benefits the liver and kidneys; the root is more useful for the liver and the leaves for the kidneys. When we discuss elder, you will find that there are different actions attributed to several different parts of the plant.

In the past few decades, a large amount of work has been done to determine just what chemical compounds in each herbs are medically useful and what actions they have. However, in practice, it is rare for herbalists to isolate individual chemical components. The herbalist's general assumption and experience is that "nature knows best" and that we meddle at our peril. We usually find that the whole combination of substances within the herb or a particular part of the herb being used is more valuable than any one component.

To illustrate this quantitatively, we can take a simple example involving a vitamin. Vitamin C is found in nearly all fruits, and these fruits confer many vitamin C-related health benefits when eaten whole. This same vitamin C can also be extracted from fruit, made into tablets, and consumed separately. However, there is a problem. By doing this, many of the other valuable compounds in the fruits, including the hundreds of different bioflavonoids, are left behind. Recent studies have shown that a group of these bioflavonoids, called oligomeric proanthocyanidins or OPCs, can increase the beneficial action of vitamin C by over 11 percent. This means that as a result of separating out the pure vitamin C, it loses over 90 percent of its effectiveness when compared to the same amount of vitamin C when consumed with the whole fruit, particularly if that fruit is rich in OPCs.

For this reason, too, you are advised to use preparations of whole herbs, or parts of herbs such as root or leaves or flowers, rather than trying to extract individual chemical ingredients.

Choosing Your Own Herbs

We will shortly be discussing a large number of herbs to help you design your own detoxification program. The Herbal Functions table is a quick reference point you can use to see which herbs perform which jobs.

Herbs have many uses and actions, and these actions or activities are given specific names. This means that it is very easy to give a quick description of an herb in only a half dozen words or less. Dandelion, for instance is a laxative, cholagogue, and diuretic. If you look below, you will discover what these words mean, although you probably know at least two of the three. There is no need to become a fully fledged herbalist to go on an herbal Detox Regime, but it will make your life easier if we list here the common functions of herbs and the meanings of the various terms. This will save having to repeat the description many times throughout the book.

Herbal Functions

DESCRIPTION	ACTION	TYPICAL HERBS
Adaptogen	helps to modulate or adjust hormonal and immune responses	cat's claw, ginseng
Alterative	blood cleanser	blue flag, burdock, echinacea, poke root, red clover, yellow dock
Analgesic Anodyne	reduces pain	black willow, cayenne, chamomile, cloves, passionflower, skullcap, valerian
Anthelmintic	acts against intestinal parasites	garlic, quassia, tansy, false unicorn root
Antiasthmatic	reduces the symptoms of asthma	lobelia, grindelia
Antibilious	reduces bile and nausea	barberry, dandelion, fringe tree, golden seal
Anticatarrhal	reduces excess catarrh	coltsfoot, echinacea, garlic, golden seal, sage, yarrow
Anticoagulant	reduces the blood's tendency to clot	cayenne, ginger, olives
Antiemetic	reduces nausea and vomiting	barberry, black horehound, meadowsweet

Antifungal	active against fungi and molds	black walnut, cinnamon, garlic, ginger, golden seal, marigold, thyme
Antihistamine	reduces the production and release of histamine	chamomile, ginger, golden root, pillbearing spurge
Anti-inflammatory	reduces inflammation	black willow, chamomile, devil's claw, St John's wort, witch hazel
Antilithic	prevents urinary stones and gravel formation	buchu, corn silk, couch grass, gravel root, pellitory of the wall, stone root
Antimicrobial	destroys or inhibits microorganisms	burdock, clove, couch grass, echinacea, eucalyptus, garlic, green tea, liquorice, myrrh, nasturtium, olive leaf, thyme, wormwood
Antineoplastic	reduces the tendency to form tumors	cat's claw, cleavers, red clover
Antioxidant	improves the body's defense against oxidizing toxins	cat's claw, cayenne, cloves, elder, ginkgo biloba, green tea, milk thistle, pine, rosemary, schizandra, turmeric
Antiscorbutic	prevents scurvy	scurvy grass, shepherd's purse, rosehip
Antiseptic	prevents putrefaction	barberry, bearberry, blessed thistle, cayenne, echinacea, garlic, golden seal, southernwood, white pond lily
Antispasmodic	reduces cramps	black haw, black cohosh, cramp bark, lady's slipper, lobelia, valerian, wild yam

Antitussive	reduces coughing	coltsfoot, elecampane
Aperient	very mild action, stimulating bowel movements	rhubarb root, dandelion, milk thistle
Aphrodisiac	sexual arousal	damiana, ginseng, saw palmetto
Aromatic	strong smell or flavor stimulates digestion	aniseed, caraway, cardamom, coriander, cumin, dill fennel, peppermint, rosemary
Astringent	tightens tissues by acting on proteins	bayberry, bistort, comfrey, eyebright, golden rod, meadowsweet, rhubarb root, St John's wort, witch hazel, yarrow
Bitter	stimulates digestion	barberry, gentian, golden seal, rhubarb root, tansy, wormwood
Cardiac tonic	benefits the heart	cayenne, cat's claw, figwort, hawthorn, lily of the valley, motherwort
Carminative	reduces flatulence	angelica, aniseed, caraway, cardamom, chamomile, dill, ginger, peppermint
Cathartic	strong evacuation	cascara sagrada, senna
Cholagogue	stimulates bile flow	balmony, barberry, blue flag, dandelion, fringe tree, milk thistle, wahoo, wild yam
Choleretic	an agent that stimulates the production of bile by the liver	gentian
Demulcent	mucilaginous, soothing, and protective	comfrey, irish moss, marsh mallow, mullein, slippery elm, milk thistle

Diaphoretic	promotes perspiration and cleansing	boneset, cayenne, garlic, ginger, guiacum, pleurisy root, prickly ash, yarrow
Diuretic	increases urination	boldo, buchu, celery seed, cleavers, corn silk, couchgrass, dandelion, gravel root, juniper, parsley piert, yarrow
Emetic	causes vomiting	ipecacuanha, lobelia (both need high doses)
Emmenagogue	normalizes menstrual flow	black cohosh, blue cohosh, false unicorn root, mugwort, penny-royal, rue, southern-wood, tansy
Emollient	softens the skin external use	chickweed, coltsfoot, comfrey, flaxseed, mallow, marsh mallow, plantain, slippery elm
Expectorant	clearing excess mucus	coltsfoot, comfrey, elecampane, grindelia, lobelia, lungwort, mullein, white hore-hound
Febrifuge	reduces fevers	cayenne, elder flower, lobelia, pennyroyal, pleurisy root
Galactagogue	stimulates flow of breast milk	aniseed, goat's rue, milk thistle
Hepatic	liver tonic	barberry, blue flag, boldo, chelidonium, dandelion, golden seal, wahoo
Hypnotic	for insomnia	hops, Jamaican dogwood, passionflower, scullcap, valerian
Hypotensive	helps normalize high blood pressure	garlic, grindelia

Laxative	stimulates bowel action	barberry, cascara sagrada, dandelion, senna, yellow dock
Nervine	benefits the nervous system	chamomile, centaury, hops, passionflower, skullcap, valerian
Oxytocic	stimulates womb contraction	blue cohosh, golden seal, squaw vine
Parasiticide	kills or removes parasites	cat's claw, aniseed rosemary
Pectoral	strengthens the respiratory system, effective in chest problems	coltsfoot, comfrey, elecampane, golden seal
Purgative	strong laxative	greater celandine, pumpkin seed, rhubarb root
Rubefacient	stimulates circulation applied externally	cayenne, ginger, horseradish, mustard
Sedative	reduces nervous tension and stress, relieves insomnia	black cohosh, hops, passionflower, skullcap, valerian
Sialagogue	stimulates saliva	cayenne, gentian
Stimulant	physiological stimulant	bayberry, cayenne, horseradish, tansy, wormwood
Tonic	toning and strengthening	agrimony, barberry, damiana, dandelion, gentian, prickly ash, wormwood
Vermifuge	eliminates worms	butternut, horehound, wormwood
Vulnerary	wound healing (external)	aloe, chickweed, comfrey, golden seal, marsh mallow, St John's wort

Herbal Preparations

Shortly we will be discussing a range of herbs in detail and in relation to the various ways they can contribute to a Detox Regime. Once you know the actions of various herbs, you can start to select the ones that will best help you. We will be discussing this in more detail later, but meanwhile, you can use the Herbal Functions table to select the herb or herbs that best cover the range of actions you want. At this point, you could make a theoretical stab at it, but I suggest you wait to decide on your final selection until we have covered the actions of the various herbs in more detail.

Once you have chosen an herb that is specific to your need, then it is time to decide in what form you are going to take it. Herbal preparations can be made in many different ways. They can be made very simply with little or no equipment, in which case they may have a very short life. You can make an herbal tea, for instance, very easily by simply adding boiling water, but it won't keep for more than a few hours.

On the other hand, they can be made by more complex methods demanding specific equipment, such as in the production of a tincture. The result is usually a remedy that will keep for a long time. There are advantages to taking herbs fresh or dried; others to taking preparations that have involved grinding, solvents, or heating processes.

Fresh Herbs

The simplest way to consume herbs is via the fresh plant. Chopped parsley on your fish, chives in your salad, or basil on your tomatoes are obvious examples. The leaves of nasturtium, dandelion, and cleavers can be added to salads; borage flowers can be used on fruit salads; nettles can be made into soup.

Herbs can be used in cooking, and you will use, or have used, culinary herbs in this way. However, you can do the same things with medicinal herbs. Many of them have little or no flavor, so they can even be "buried" or hidden within your food and escape your notice. There could hardly be an easier way of taking a remedy.

There are many advantages to using fresh herbs. Ideally, grow your own. Then pick them fresh and consume them within a short time of picking. In this way, the vital energies and delicate components are maintained at maximum concentration. Some vitamins, for instance, break down gradually with time, and with a variety of treatments. The sooner you eat them the better.

There are also disadvantages to taking herbs in this way. Some of the active ingredients are very firmly bound within the plant's cells, or complexed with some of the indigestible parts of the herb. These may, when eaten, be passed through your system and not absorbed. A preparation in which heat is applied or the active ingredients are extracted into alcohol can often get around this problem.

No matter where you live, you can grow herbs. If you have a garden of any size, you can grow herbs, and there are countless books available to tell you how. If you only have a terrace, balcony, or other concrete surface, you can still grow herbs. Grow them in pots, grow bags, or other suitable containers. If you have no flat surface, grow them vertically. Grow them from hanging baskets. Alternatively, it is a simple matter to make a firm wooden framework of horizontal and vertical struts. Fix this securely to a wall. Then lash, clamp, or tie each pot to the framework and plant them up. In this way you should be able to grow quite a large number of herbs on a wall space of only, for instance, ten square feet. Grow them in window boxes. Grow them indoors as well as outside. Most of them make interesting, beautiful, and often aromatic potted plants.

When they are at their most productive, don't forget to harvest them. Cut off as much as you choose and dry this surplus so you have a ready source during the winter months.

Dried Herbs

Dried herbs offer some advantages. There is the obvious one of convenience. You are not dependent on a fresh supply. Dried herbs can be stored, almost indefinitely, although in general you should aim to replace last year's stocks with the new season's harvest. Unlike fresh herbs, you are more likely to use the whole plant, the stems as well as the leaves. Another is that they can be ground until extremely fine. This process breaks down as many of the structures as possible, the seed, leaf, or stem structure, as well as that of the individual cells. In this way, the constituents are made more available for easy processing in your digestive system and easy absorption.

Drying herbs is a simple matter, and there are several ways of doing it. A traditional one with a wonderful image of old-fashioned country cottages, is to hang them in bunches, from the rafters, or, more prosaically, from a convenient hook. The problem with this method is that they gather dust in the process. If you have a *very* cool warming oven, they can be laid on trays and dried in it. It is generally best to leave the door open and allow many hours for gentle drying. Using the main oven is not a good idea, as it is all too easy to burn the herbs. In any case, long and slow drying is best. You may find that you already have a suitably warm space in your house. Your linen cupboard may house the hot-water tank and thus provide an appropriately warm and dust-free space. Your water heater may be housed in a cupboard with a suitable space, either above or below it, to place trays of herbs. Beside the heat vent at the back of your refrigerator may be a suitable place. Alternatively, you might decide to take this very seriously and buy yourself a drying oven, specifically designed for drying herbs and other foods.

The dried herbs can be used in the same way as fresh ones. You can add them to salad dressing and to cooking generally. You can also use them to make an herb salt. Buying herb salt is generally a costly business, you pay a high price for adding a small amount of herb to the very inexpensive salt. Making your own is simple, very inexpensive, and you can dictate the ingredients you want. You may even choose to have a variety of herbal salts. Some of them might be purely for flavor; others might be for specific medicinal purposes. To make them, all you need is some salt and the herb or herbs you want. If you are making the salt for flavor, combine the herbs and the salt in the proportions that suit your palette. If using them for medicinal purposes, then use a minimum of salt to get the maximum benefit.

First dry the herbs. Then you will need some means of grinding them. You can use a pestle and mortar, a small electrical coffee grinder, or a blender or food processor. Combine the dried herbs and the salt, blend, and it's done. Store them in an airtight jar. They look attractive in glass jars on open shelves, although they may keep slightly longer if stored in the dark. Wherever you store them, make sure they are easily available. If you have to go some distance from the stove, you are as likely to grab for the plain salt as for one of your own special herbal preparations.

Dried Herbs in Capsules Another way to take dried herbal preparations is in capsules. Empty capsules, of several sizes, can generally be bought from chemists and then filled by hand. This is easily done. Simply hold the top and bottom of the capsule in each hand, bring the two together through a pile of the powdered herb, and close the capsule. Small gadgets are also available for doing this. You simply sit the capsule bases into the hollows in a horizontal tray, brush the powdered herb over the top (rather like filling an ice cube tray with water), then place the capsule tops in the holes in the gadget lid, place the lid over the base, and press. There you have it, twenty or more filled and closed capsules.

You can, of course, also buy the capsule already prepared. Your health-food store almost certainly stocks a wide range of herbal preparations in dry capsule form. These may be individual herbs, such as echinacea or milk thistle, or they may be combinations of herbs aimed at a specific health problem.

Give some thought to what the capsule is made of. Typically gelatin capsules are used. But you can also get capsules made from plant sources. This may be important if you are vegetarian or concerned for any other reason about eating such animal-based products.

Dried Herbs in Pellet Form You can make the dried herb into pellets or pills using a variety of foods. This is particularly useful when you are dealing with children who may dislike swallowing capsules or tablets. Although I'm not normally an advocate of white bread, in this instance it can be useful. You probably remember making bread pellets at school as you rolled the crumbs between finger and thumb. This time you simply combine the crumbled fresh bread with the dried herbs and roll the two together and shape into a pellet. These pellets are soft and easily swallowed. Other foods can be used for the same purpose. Peanut butter or cream cheese combine well with the herbal powder and form discrete pellets. Or mix the herbs with honey and take from a teaspoon.

Lozenges Lozenges are surprisingly simple to make and are an excellent way to take an herbal mixture when you want something to suck for a mouth problem or to soothe a sore throat. You will need a source of mucilage such as slippery elm or marsh mallow powder, or a gum such as tragacanth. If you use tragacanth, soak ¼ cup in water for 24 hours, stirring frequently. Then add it to two cups of boiling water. Mix thoroughly until smooth and then press through a muslin sieve. Add the powdered dried herbs or the essential oils of the desired herbs, sugar (if you feel you must), roll out on a cold surface dusted with cornflour to prevent sticking, cut into shapes, and allow to dry. Once made, the lozenges should be stored in an airtight container.

Alternatively, you can use gelatin. Make the jelly, with water, in the usual way, but using less water to make a firmer product than you would do for a dessert. Add the herbs, again either in the dried form or as the essential oils, pour into a flat dish, allow to cool, then cut and store.

Liquid Preparations

There are several different liquid herbal preparations that you can make at home. They include the use of water, vinegars, oils, glycerine, sugar, or alcohol. As a general guide, infusions are made by pouring the liquid on the herbs and allowing the mixture to stand for a period of time that can extend from a few minutes to days, weeks, or even years.

For herbs that are hard and woody, for stems, roots, and even some seeds, decoctions offer more benefits than infusions. Decoctions involve boiling or simmering the herbs in the chosen liquid.

Water-based Infusions Water-based herbal preparations are either infusions or decoctions. Infusions are made in the same way as an everyday cup of tea. Boil the water and pour it over the fresh or dried herb in a cup or teapot, and allow it to infuse for a few minutes.

Ideally, infusions should be made in china or glassware. Do not use a metal teapot, and particularly not an aluminium one. Alternatively, put the herb in a special double spoon designed for the purpose. It will have holes through the top and bottom so the hot water can soak the herb and extract many of the active ingredients. You can also use bamboo or similar containers with holes punched through them, available from many Chinese shops. Infusions can be made with fresh or dried herbs. You will need about three times as much of the fresh herb as the dried herb. The usual amounts are one teaspoonful of dried herb or three of fresh to one cup of water. Allow the herb to steep for about fifteen minutes before drinking. Infusions can be drunk hot or cold. They are best made from the softer parts of the herb, the leaves, or flowers. To make an infusion from the seeds, stem, bark, or roots, it is best to grind the herb first, as finely as possible, to ensure maximum extraction of the active ingredients.

Some herbs are sensitive to heat. Others contain aromatic oils that could be lost when heated; others contain ingredients that are heat-sensitive and might break down. Both these groups of herbs can be made into cold infusions. Simply add the cold water to the herb and allow to steep in a sealed container for twelve hours or overnight. If the herb contains aromatic oils and you really do want to take it hot, make the infusion in a pot with a tight lid on to retain as much of the aromatic oil as possible.

Infusions are obviously the basis of many herb teas. You can now buy teas made from a wide range of herbs. They may consist of a single herb or a combination of herbs. Many of them include fruit extracts for added flavor. If the herbal tea that you want, for therapeutic reasons, does not appeal to your taste buds, try combining it with one that does, such as peppermint. Herbal teas can be bought as tea bags or as the loose herb.

Flowers and leaves make the best infusions. Consider some of these:

Alfalfa	good for arthritis, often combined with peppermint for flavor
Chamomile	to relax, physically and mentally, and to improve digestion
Elder flower	good for clearing out the toxins of a cold and breaking up the catarrh, also has a pleasant flavor
Hyssop	can help to clear chronic catarrh

Peppermint	does wonders for a blocked head cold or sluggish digestion
Red Clover	a good blood cleanser, good for your skin and lungs and with a delicate and pleasing flavor
Rosemary	can help to clear parasites from your digestive tract
Sage	swirl it as a mouthwash, too, for bleeding or infected gums
Thyme	a useful antiseptic, for sore throats and catarrh, helpful in dealing with parasites
Valerian	for a good night's sleep

Glycerine-Based Infusions Glycerine, possibly more familiar as the sweet liquid or glycerol used to make cake icing, can be used to extract some of the herb's components. Glycerine is a better solvent than water for many of the herbal constituents, though not as good as alcohol. However, it is often a preferred option if you want something stronger than the water extract but don't want, for whatever reason, to use alcohol.

Glycerine comes from fat. The vast majority of the fats you eat, be they animal fats or vegetable oils, are triglycerides. You may have heard of them in relation to blood tests, as they are the compounds that are measured in your blood, together with cholesterol, when your blood fats are being measured.

Triglycerides are made from three fatty acids (hence, the tri-) added to one unit of glycerol (glyceride). Although glycerol comes from and is part of the fats in your diet, on its own, glycerol is actually a sweet and slightly sticky liquid.

When making an herbal infusion, use a 50-50 mixture of glycerine and water. Use about ½ cup of dried herb or 1 cup of the fresh herb and add to a mixture of ¼ cup of glycerine and ¼ cup of water. Let the mixture infuse, in a stoppered container, for two or three weeks, shaking it a few times each day. Then strain, wring out to extract the last of the liquid, store the liquid, and use as needed.

Glycerine has another excellent use. On its own it makes an excellent and extremely cheap hand cream. To use it, first wash your hands, then, with clean but wet hands, apply a few drops of glycerine, rub all over, and towel dry. You will need a specific towel for this, as it does get rather sticky with use. If you do this each time you wash your hands, they will become wonderfully soft.

Alcohol-and-Water-Based Infusions There is another very pleasant way to make infusions and that is to soak the herb in alcohol. The alcohol could be wine, sherry, or one of the spirits such as vodka or brandy. Sloe gin is an early and well-known example of this method. Sloes are allowed to sit in a bottle of gin until the gin has acquired much of the flavor and some of the benefits of the sloes. You can then truly say you are just having a medicinal drink. Such infusions are the historical basis for tonic wines, aperitifs, and liqueurs.

If you use wine to make the infusion, the resultant tonic will not keep, so drink it within a few days. This is for two reasons. First, there is insufficient alcohol in the wine to act as a long-term preservative; and second, the wine will still oxidize at its normal rate. For a preparation that lasts longer, you can use a fortified wine such as sherry or port. Ginger wine, still commercially available, is a good example of this.

Since enjoyment is a component of this method of taking herbs, you will want to experiment with combinations and quantities that give off a pleasing flavor. A good tonic to start with would be one to aid and normalize your digestive system. Try a mixture of such stomach-calming herbs (carminatives) as peppermint, ginger, cumin, cardamom, anise, and fennel. If you suspect you have parasites, add rosemary, thyme, or wormwood. Allow these to steep in the wine for an hour or two before drinking, or add them to your current bottle of sherry or port.

If you become a real enthusiast, you could ferment your own herbs, turning them into a variety of homemade wines. Most people have heard of elderberry wine, dandelion wine, and others. Although most of the alcohol in these is derived from the sugar used, many of the active and beneficial compounds in the herbs seep into the wine during the course of their manufacture.

Alcohol-Based Infusions — Tinctures In general usage, an infusion is taken to mean a water, wine, or oil-based preparation of an herb. When the herbal ingredients are extracted into strong alcohol, the resultant liquid is generally called a tincture.

As we have seen, the components of many herbs are not soluble in water. Some are not soluble in the weak alcohol-water mixture, that is wine, nor do they keep so well that way. The solution to this is either to consume the herb whole or to dissolve the constituents in some other liquid in which these components are soluble.

Many of the active ingredients of herbs will dissolve in strong alcohol. Not only that, but alcohol has another advantage over water on its own or the weaker alcohol and water mixture of wine. Alcohol, when present in sufficient strength, acts as a preservative, and any preparation made with it can be kept for an extended period.

Many of the herbal preparations you buy in the stores in liquid form are alcoholic tinctures. When these are made, there are generally very specific guidelines as to the exact amount of each herb and the exact proportions of the liquids; they are made to pre-determined standards so you know what you are getting. They may also have been heated during preparation.

When you make your own at home, such exactness is not required. Thus, the procedure is very much simplified.

To make your own alcohol-based herbal tincture:

i Put three cups of dried herb or four cups of fresh herb in a large container with a tight-fitting lid. A large jar will do. The ones used for bottling fruit are excellent. It should not have a metallic lid.
ii Add two cups of 60% proof vodka or brandy.
iii Close the container, put in a warm place, and shake the mixture two or three times a day for two or three weeks.
iv Strain through a muslin cloth, wringing out the last drops of the liquid, as they contain valuable ingredients.
v The liquid can be stored in tightly stoppered bottles, and the leftover solids will do wonders for your potted plants.

Herbalists generally recommend from ten drops to a teaspoon of a tincture up to three times a day. Remember that tinctures are a lot stronger than infusions or decoctions. They can be taken neat, or with water or fruit juice.

Oil-Based Infusions Herbs can be allowed to steep in oils, such as olive oil, that will later be used in cooking or in salad dressings.

Fill an empty bottle with the selected herb or herbs. Add the very best virgin olive oil you can get, preferably organic. Seal, and allow to steep for a month. Strain off the oil, pressing the herbs thoroughly, and store the oil in an airtight bottle. Use as desired. The residual herbs can also be added to cooking, if appropriate. It is best not to leave the herbs in the oil, as eventually, as the oil is used, they become exposed above the oil level. Bacteria and other organisms can then grow on them, and the oil can be affected.

Vinegar-Based Infusions Another culinary infusion involves the use of vinegar. You may have already used tarragon vinegar, made by steeping a sprig of tarragon in a bottle of vinegar. You can buy these herbal vinegars, and pay a lot of money for them, or you can make them yourself.

Simply choose the herbs you want to use, put them in a bottle, add the vinegar, and allow the mixture to steep for a week or two. The best vinegar to use is apple cider vinegar, as it has health benefits of its own. You could also use a pure wine vinegar. Avoid the commercial vinegars that are little more than bottles of diluted acetic acid. As you use the vinegar, the level will eventually fall below that of the herb. When this happens, remove the exposed herb, otherwise it can go moldy and affect the rest of the mixture.

Water-Based Decoctions The simplest decoctions are made, like simple infusions, by the simple addition of water, the difference being that in this instance the mixture is heated to increase the release of the soluble components into the water. Use the same quantities as before, one teaspoon of the dried herb or two or three teaspoons of the fresh herb to each cup of water. Chop and/or grind the herb as finely as possible before adding the water. Use a stainless steel or glass saucepan, not one made from aluminium. If the herb contains valuable volatile oils, put a lid on the pan, although it is generally better to grind them exceedingly fine and make an infusion instead. Simmer for about ten to fifteen minutes and then strain while hot.

Alcohol-Based Decoctions Herbal decoctions can also be made using alcohol and the mixture heated, but this, to be generally effective, requires special equipment.

Improving the Flavor

Many herbal preparations taste fine, you only have to think of the culinary herbs and spices to recognize how enjoyable many of them can be. Herbs are generally added to food *purely* for their flavor, although you may also make some of the choices on medical grounds. Likewise, most people who choose to drink herbal teas do enjoy the flavor of them on their own. Others prefer to add honey to sweeten the brew. This is a shame, as neither honey nor sugar provide any beneficial nutrients on their own; they provide caloric energy without any of the vitamins and minerals needed to extract and use this energy properly. However, if the honey is needed to make the herbal tea the drink of choice rather than coffee, it is probably the lesser of the two evils, and at least you are also getting the benefit of the herb.

If, on the other hand, you are using the herb sage tea or thyme tea for instance, as a gargle when you have oral thrush and a sore throat, the honey can add a soothing dimension. Honey is also useful when giving infusions to young children who have already acquired a sweet tooth as a result of previous habits. Note, however, that if your baby has colic and you give him chamomile tea, he will generally take it quite happily without the honey. After all, to babies all experiences are new, and this is just one new experience. They do not yet have any preconceived expectations of sweetness in what they drink.

However, in general the tinctures of most medicinal herbs have a strong taste and one that is rarely to people's liking. The purists and the brave will simply hold their breath and drink down the mixture, possibly having something pleasant-tasting at hand afterwards to take the taste away. For the faint-hearted, there are other possibilities.

Herbal tinctures can be made more palatable by combining them with honey or a sugar syrup. There are several ways of doing this.

For mild-tasting tinctures, use the following method to make a syrup. Combine two cups of water with four cups of sugar, heat until it dissolves and stir thoroughly until a syrup is formed. This can then be combined in equal parts with the tincture.

Another way to hide the taste is to use a mixture of honey and apple cider vinegar. Combine four parts of honey with one part of apple cider vinegar, and heat until it forms a syrup. If you are making your own preparation from strongly flavored herbs, you can add the herbs to this mixture and heat until a combined syrup is formed. The proportions of the honey-vinegar mix to the herb will depend on the extent to which you wish to hide the flavor of the latter. Use as little of the honey mixture as you can to make the taste tolerable. If you are starting with a purchased tincture, combine this tincture with as little of the honey-vinegar mixture as you can to suit your taste buds.

Availability of Herbs and Dosage

Grow Your Own

I've already mentioned growing your own, and in the final section of this book, you will find a chapter devoted specifically to herbs whose the seeds are readily available from gardening suppliers (p.278).

Supermarkets

You will find many beneficial herbs on the kitchen shelves in supermarkets. There is a growing tendency to supply pots of fresh herbs as well as packets of fresh herbs, and of course you can buy them as dried herbs. It is no coincidence that most of the spices used in curries are carminatives and help to relieve flatulence. If you exclude chilli or cayenne itself, none of them are "hot;" they are simply the seeds of herbal plants. There is a special chapter devoted to the medicinal uses of culinary herbs (p.236).

Health-Food Stores

Many herbs can be found in the herbal tea sections of supermarkets and health-food stores. Health-food stores also carry a range of herbs as tablets, capsules, or tinctures. Some of them consist of single herbs; others are compounded of several herbs all with a similar or complementary action and often designed for a specific purpose.

Specialty Herbal Suppliers

Less common herbs are available from specialty herbal shops, many of which will supply them by mail order.

Throughout this book, I have, where possible, referred to and included herbs that are readily available in supermarkets, food, and health-food stores. However, I have not hesitated to refer to other herbs as well when they provide valuable benefits. There are many excellent books available on herbs and herbal medicine to which you can refer if you wish to learn more.

Dosage and How Much to Take

In Part IV, individual herbs are described in connection with parts of the body, and dosage details are given such that you can use the fresh or dried herb. Thus there are descriptions for making either the infusion or the decoction. There are also dosages for the tinctures, in case you buy these instead. It is important to recognize, however, that purchased tinctures can vary in strength, and if the manufacturer's dosage is different from the one given here, then you should follow it.

The dosage for each herb is given in the section that includes the main description of that herb — not every time the herb is mentioned. If you cannot find the dosage in a particular section, go to the index and look for the page indicated in bold type.

You may prefer to purchase the herbs as tablets or capsules, in which case follow the recommended dosage on the label.

Choosing a Multiple Remedy

You may find that you are purchasing a supplement with more than one herb in it. When selecting a multiple herbal remedy, you may find a number of different preparations all purporting to achieve the aim you are after. There may be, for instance, several preparations to help your liver or improve the quality of your skin. They will all list the different herbs that are included. By considering the information given in Part IV, you will be able to make a more secure selection based on the product that contains the herbs that best covers your needs.

Restrictions to Supplies

There is a growing tendency in some countries to restrict the sale and availability of herbal preparations. This is allegedly connected with safety issues. However, there is negligible evidence that herbal remedies can do you harm, certainly in comparison with the multitude of over-the-counter medicines. The damage done by these makes the mis-use of herbal remedies minor by comparison, if not non-existant. In fact, the restrictions proposed for the UK, for example, are becoming draconian and could very well mean that you have to be particularly inventive to obtain the remedy you are after. However, do persist, for the results will certainly be worth the effort.

Progressively, herbs are being removed from the list of those that can be purchased. The situation is being made worse by the increasing requirements the government is imposing on the manufacturing companies, requirements so costly that no company could hope to get its money back on products that cannot, by their nature, be patented. This, to say the least, is a great shame. It is also very wrong, in the view of many, to restrict the avenues to health that are available to the individual and to leave them with few options but the use of chemical drugs with toxic side effects.

There are other considerations. For every person who treats and heals him- or herself with herbs, there is one less person who depends on state medical systems for treatment, and there is one less person in danger of suffering from the side effects that all medical drugs produce. This, you might think, would be a persuasive point for governments who are perennially faced with the increased cost of providing health care to the nation. However, the forces of the large multinational pharmaceutical companies and other vested interests seem to be more powerful.

Fortunately, many herbal preparations are now available over the Internet, and this should be treated as a valuable resource. We are not able to provide a full list here, which would be so vast that it would need a separate book in itself and is, in any case, growing continually. So do some research for yourself. At the time of going to press, **www.herbalmedicine.com** can almost certainly lead you to what you want.

The proposed restrictions on the domestic supply of medicinal herbs makes the knowledge of what culinary herbs can do all the more important. It also means that growing your own may be one way you can take care of your health and that we may witness a return to the old ways, when the wild plants of the garden and countryside were common components of the medical chest.

✦✦✦   ✦✦✦

PART IV

Your Body's Systems — Which Herbs to Use

✦✦✦

RIGHT, SO YOU'VE TIDIED UP YOUR HOME and workplace. You've eliminated as many sources of toxins as you can. You've learned something about herbs in general. Now it is time to get down to business, to focus on your body as it is at the moment and how you can take care of it from now on. It is time to learn about the various ways of getting rid of the toxins that are already within your system. It is time to learn about ways of preventing new toxins, the ones you cannot avoid, from being absorbed. And it is time to learn about specific herbs and what they can do for you, for your own particular needs and state of health.

We will start with elimination. Your four-week Detox Regime will include the herbs to help you eliminate the toxins stored in your body. What you will learn in this section is which herbs can help in the elimination of toxins as an ongoing process. You will recall that there are four main areas or ways via which toxins can be eliminated from your body — namely, via the digestive system in the feces; via the kidneys in urine; via the lungs in expelled air and sputum; and via the skin. These four systems need to be supported so they can do their job to the fullest.

You can prevent the absorption of toxins from your digestive tract by not eating or drinking foods laden with toxic chemicals. However, you cannot always eat organic foods, and you cannot avoid all toxins. So it is important to ensure that, if you do ingest toxins, they are not absorbed from your digestive tract into your bloodstream. Herbs can help.

We will be considering the particular herbs that contribute to normal and healthy digestion and ensure good digestive function. We will be considering herbs that help to prevent putrefaction and a buildup of new toxins within the gut, and we will be looking at herbs that ensure proper bowel function and prevent constipation, thus aiding the rapid elimination of waste material. We will be considering herbs that help your liver to function its best, as this plays a major role in the body's efforts to eliminate toxins from within the system. We will also be considering herbs that help to prevent damage to the lining of your digestive tract, as any such damage could facilitate the absorption of toxins from your gut into your bloodstream. Symptoms such as altered bowel function or the presence of mucus, suggest that toxins are being eliminated through the digestive system. Help is needed to encourage and complete this process.

Similarly, we will be considering herbs that help the elimination of excess mucus from the lungs; and herbs that facilitate normal lung function and that can be used in situations where lung, bronchial, or nasal tissues are infected or damaged, such as with bronchitis or sinusitis.

Infections of the kidneys or urinary tract can interfere with normal elimination, so we will be considering herbs that can correct a variety of problems in these areas. Cystitis needs treatment for its own sake, as does thrush, otherwise there can be a buildup of toxins. Fluid buildup in the body can hinder elimination and so, where needed, diuretic herbs will be helpful. We will be discussing these.

Any sign of ill health in the skin could be a sign that a Detox Regime is needed. Gray skin, dull skin that has lost its glow and and dark shadows under the eyes can all be a sign of ill health and toxic overload. The gray shadows under the eyes are often associated with liver or kidney problems. Pimples, acne, boils, or other signs of skin infections call for the various herbs that can help to eliminate the associated toxins from your body. Cuts, grazes, burns, or any other type of wound requires treatment with herbs to help the healing process and eliminate the chance of toxins entering your bloodstream or the wound becoming infected. Dry skin or itchy rashes are signs that your skin is not in good health and help is needed.

It is also important to have a fully functioning immune system. Your white blood cells must be able to recognize foreign bodies, attack them, and either break them down or package them into a form such that they can be safely transported through your bloodstream and out, usually via your liver or kidneys. Your antigens and the various other components of your immune system must all be functioning at their best. Any signs of inflammation can mean that there are toxins present that your body is trying to isolate, break down, and eliminate. This process should be supported, and a resolution sought as soon as possible. Thus, we will be considering a range of herbs that will help your immune system.

Your lymphatic system, a transport system somewhat analogous to a parallel bloodstream, though with some important differences, is responsible for gathering up toxins from the various parts of your body and delivering them to the exit routes. On the way, they will pass your various lymph nodes and glands. If these become swollen, painful, or infected, then it is important to provide support for their proper function to hasten the Detox process. So we will be considering a number of herbs that can be of assistance.

The bloodstream itself can become laden with toxins. Alterative herbs are also known as "blood cleansers," and these are important herbs to consider.

I have already mentioned the liver as being an important player in the Detox process within your digestive system. It is also important systemically, from inside your body. Once toxins are released from wherever they are being stored, or once they have been digested and transported through the blood, they eventually reach the liver, and it is the job of this organ to package them in a form such that they can do minimal harm.

So in the following chapters, we will be looking at all these topics in much greater detail and considering the various herbs that can help. I have focused on herbs that play these specific roles. However, it is normal to find that a blood cleanser or a liver herb may also benefit some other organ such as the heart, or be useful in dealing with some other health problem such as rheumatism. Where appropriate, I have mentioned these actions, since you may well be suffering from some of these conditions and could choose an herb that will both perform the specific Detox action you want and help some other problem you may have. You might as well get the double benefit if it is possible. This means that, although we may seem to be ranging far and wide with the herbs discussed, the main focus of each of them is still on detoxing your body in whatever way is most useful to you.

I have intentionally not included herbs whose main role is in the treatment of such problems as heart disease, although cleaning up the arteries could possibly, if the definition was extended, be considered a Detox Regime. Nor have I considered herbs whose main role is in dealing with arthritis, diabetes, or any of a number of health problems that are not directly immediate problems of toxins.

To avoid confusion, I have tried to give the Latin names for all the herbs as well as their common name. This will help if you are trying to obtain the herbs in or from other countries.

I have listed the actions of the herbs in their more technical and brief forms, but if you forget the meaning of one of the actions, refer to the Herbal Functions table on p.57.

Keep in mind that many of the herbs are common and are found in the garden or in the kitchen. Use these herbs whenever possible. You can always make them into teas or add them to cooking, and many of them will become part of an appropriate prevention program. Eat garlic dishes with thyme and sage for a range of antiparasitic effects; use red clover flowers to make an excellent blood cleansing tea; use herbs such as peppermint or cumin to relieve flatulence and improve digestion. Many of the herbs can be included in salads as well as flavorings, such as the leaves of nasturtium, dandelion, sorrel, and others. Make a practice of doing this. You may choose to start off with one or two at a time, then gradually increase your repertoire.

Your diet is also important. Include as many fresh fruits, vegetables, salads, and herbs as possible. Many such foods can help the detox process. Some can do this actively. Onions and garlic, for instance, act against a variety of parasites, as do herbs such as sage and thyme. Other vegetables give you valuable nutrients to support your immune system or to provide the liver with nutrients it needs to deal with toxins.

I hope I have included sufficient folklore and history to bring the herbs to light and give a clear picture of what they can accomplish. At the end of the day, the choice is yours. Use the information in the following chapters to select herbs that will help you to improve your overall health in the specific ways that you require. Keep in mind, all the time, that while you are selecting your own Detox Regime, prevention is easier than cure, so clean up your act.

+ + +   + + +

✦ CHAPTER 8 ✦

Your Digestive Tract

AS YOU READ THIS CHAPTER, remember that your digestive tract is a tube some 35 feet long that runs through your body. However, it is also more than that. It is certainly the place where digestion takes place. It is also a surface through which a range of substances are both absorbed and eliminated. It is the major interface between your body and the rest of the world. In area, it is about 100 times greater than the area of your skin.

Your digestive tract is the home of a vast number of microorganisms; in fact, there are more organisms there than there are cells in the rest of your body. Some of these organisms are harmful, some are or could be beneficial, and many of them are neither — they simply find it a convenient place to reside. It has often been said that many of them are very beneficial, making a number of essential vitamins and other compounds that we then absorb and use for ourselves. However, other research seems to indicate that, while they do indeed make a variety of vitamins, most of these are for their own use. Some of them may even utilize the vitamins we ingest for ourselves. The fact remains, they are there, and we need to ensure that we encourage the best of them and keep the harmful ones out.

Many factors have to come into play before your digestive system can function properly. The sight, smell, and anticipated taste of foods play a role, via a number of nerve stimuli. The evoked memories of foods also act on the brain and affect your response to foods, and both your nervous and your hormone systems come into play. This web of nerves can be called an enteric (gut-related) nervous system, and can either act largely independently of the brain or be closely interrelated with the brain. You are probably aware of this close connection between brain and digestion. When you are cross or upset, anxious or nervous, the first system that is affected is commonly your gut, as you feel nauseated, experience diarrhea or lose your appetite altogether.

Your digestive system is your first line of defense. If toxins enter this system or tube but can be eliminated before they are absorbed into your bloodstream, you have saved yourself from further potential damage. Your digestive tract is a major entry route for toxins; it is also a major elimination route. Further, if there are problems within your digestive system, you can actually create toxins in situ that can then be absorbed into your bloodstream and so transported throughout your body, something you should try to avoid at all costs.

Do you suffer from bad breath, coated tongue, sore or bleeding gums, frequent sore throats, burping, indigestion, heartburn, stomach or duodenal ulcers, flatulence or bloating, diarrhea or constipation, irritable bowel syndrome, abdominal pain or cramping, hemorrhoids, or any other disorder of your digestive tract? If so, then improving your digestive function and healing any problem area should be a first step in your detoxification program. There are several reasons for this.

- Your entire digestive tract is lined by mucilaginous material that is designed to protect the muscular walls, from your mouth and esophagus at the top, to your colon at the other end. This protection starts with the saliva you produce in your mouth and continues with the mucus produced by the mucous membranes all the way through.
- Your stomach, which contains the very strong hydrochloric acid that is so important for your digestion, is lined with a particularly strong mucous lining. If there is any damage to any part of this lining then, in addition to all the other problems that can arise such as ulcers and pain, toxins can enter.
- If you are not producing sufficient saliva, mucus, hydrochloric acid, or digestive enzymes, then food, including allergens and some toxins, will not be broken down properly and may be absorbed intact into your bloodstream. You may also fail to absorb essential nutrients, and so your overall health and detox capacity will be diminished.
- When digestion is slow, then food can start to ferment, new compounds — many of them toxic — are created, and these can be absorbed.

- The abnormal environment created by poor digestion encourages the growth of unwanted organisms which can, in turn, also produce compounds that are toxic to you and yet may be absorbed into your system.
- If you are constipated and the undigested food remains for too long in your colon, further fermentation can occur — further production of toxins that can, in turn, be absorbed into your bloodstream.

Constipation is a lot more common than is generally recognized. In fact, I would say there are very few people in this country who are not constipated. The proper frequency for bowel movements is three times a day, or as often as you eat. You only have to think about it to see the logic of that. Each time you eat, there is a new quantity of food going down the tube, being digested and then waiting for elimination. If two of these food masses have to wait for the third, for the one daily exit, then fermentation and problems will inevitably occur. If you go even less than once a day, the problems are correspondingly compounded.

What's more, the stool should be soft — "mushy" being an appropriate if not very technical term. Countless patients have told me that soon after improving their diet, they have developed diarrhea, yet when they are questioned further, it turns out their motions are merely normalizing. The hard lumps we take as normal are not. The easy passage of a soft (not liquid) stool constitutes normal elimination and inhibits the formation of new toxins. Generally, in dealing with constipation, the focus should be on gentle bulking agents (including herbs), not on strong laxative and cathartic ones. We will be discussing this further, and the ways to achieve it, when we consider individual herbs.

Many systemic toxins are eliminated from your body via your liver and gallbladder, through your small intestine, and then along your colon on their way out. You do not want to have them hanging about in this lower part of your digestive tract waiting for delayed elimination. So two things are important here: first, the function of your liver and gallbladder in ensuring their efficient elimination from your bloodstream; and, second, the function of your intestines and the efficient elimination of these toxins from your colon. We will start at the top of your digestive tract.

Herbs to Make Your Mouth Water

The proper flow of saliva is an essential trigger to stimulate the rest of your digestive system into action. As increased amounts of saliva enter the stomach, this organ is alerted to the probable arrival of food and the production of stomach acid, and other digestive juices is stimulated. Conversely, this is one of the reasons why chewing gum is not good for you. The action of chewing the gum fools the stomach, for a while anyway, into thinking that food is coming down and will have to be dealt with. However, this over-stimulated release of stomach acid can in the end lead to exhaustion. The cells that produce the acid become worn out and the production of acid is reduced, even when the trigger is real and food is being eaten. This can then lead to further digestive problems in a domino effect.

Saliva includes substances that protect the lining of your mouth and help to hold the food together in one mass. If you have ever tried to eat something when your mouth is dry, you will know how difficult it is to get it all to the back of your mouth and swallowed. It keeps moving around, refusing to go down. And a glass of water doesn't help. It needs the sticky mucus to meld the chewed food into a ball ready for easy swallowing.

Saliva also contains a number of digestive enzymes, particularly ones that break carbohydrates down into simple disaccharides or double sugars (two single sugars, such as glucose, joined together). Unfortunately, some of the work of these enzymes is wasted as few people chew their food sufficiently to give the enzymes time to do their job before the food reaches the acid of the stomach, where these enzymes cease to be active. So the old adage remains true, chew your food thoroughly before you attempt to swallow it.

A number of herbs can be used to stimulate the flow of saliva, and these are called *sialagogues*. They include cayenne (as you will know from eating curries), ginger, licorice, tamarind (a fruit often used in curries), and turkey rhubarb root.

In general, they all have a similar effect on the digestive system. They differ, however, in the other properties they have. Several factors will help to dictate which one you choose. You may base your choice of individual herb on availability. Or it may be that you can purchase a combination remedy that contains more than one of them. The best method is to choose the one that has other activities that suit your own particular situation and state of overall health. You will learn which herbs can do this for you in this Part of the book.

Cayenne

Cayenne is the cayenne pepper or red chili that is used in curries. Its Latin name is *Capsicum minimum,* indicating both its relationship to other capsicums or peppers and its size. It comes from the *Solanaceae* family that also includes potatoes and tomatoes.

Cayenne pepper is made by harvesting the fruits when fully ripe, allowing them to dry in the shade and then grinding them to a powder.

Cayenne has a number of roles. It is an antiseptic, carminative, rubefacient, sialogogue, stimulant, and tonic. It is a very useful local stimulant and tonic. It scavenges or "mops up" free radicals or oxidizing agents such as singlet oxygen; thus, it is an antioxidant and can protect against the damage done by oxidizing agents and free radicals. You will find an explanation of the importance of antioxidants later on.

Cayenne helps to reduce the formation of unwanted blood clots and to normalize blood flow. This offers many benefits. It can help to stimulate circulation in cases of cold hands and feet and chilblains, and has been found to be useful in the prevention of migraines if these are caused by restricted blood flow to the brain. As an analgesic, it helps to control pain.

It can stimulate the immune system and help to ward off colds and influenza. For sore throats and laryngitis, it can be used as a gargle, and for this purpose it combines well with myrrh, which is soothing.

It can even be used externally, with caution. Applying a poultice of it can help relieve the pain of lumbago and rheumatism. It can also be used on unbroken chilblains to stimulate the circulation. But be careful — if you use it on broken skin you will soon know all about it.

For our Detox purposes, it stimulates the flow of both saliva and gastric secretions from the stomach, including hydrochloric acid and digestive enzymes, thus stimulating and improving digestion. It's useful in the treatment of flatulence, dyspepsia, and colic. And it helps to soothe the mucous membranes lining the digestive tract.

This latter statement may seem surprising since the popular expectation is that chili will irritate the digestive tract. Keep in mind, however, that there is *supposed* to be very strong acid in the stomach, that the stomach lining is ideally prepared for and protected from the effects of this acid, and that most digestive problems stem, in whole or in part, from a *lack* of stomach acid. There are almost no reported and fully confirmed cases of problems caused by an *excess* of stomach acid. Some years ago when I was in practice in Sydney, Australia, the local hospital, at great expense, imported equipment from England to measure stomach acid levels. They were looking for a correlation between stomach and duodenal ulcers and a raised output of hydrochloric acid in the stomach. They apparently didn't find a single case. Unfortunately, they did not investigate the possibility that the people concerned were suffering from low levels of stomach acid and did not look for this.

Furthermore, an interesting experiment was done many years ago, reported by nutrition writer Adelle Davis. It involved a man with both a stomach ulcer and a fistula. The latter meant that a tube could be inserted into his stomach and researchers could observe the effect of different foods on his stomach lining and the state of his ulcer. To their surprise, they found that cayenne not only did not inflame the ulcer, but that in fact it seemed to soothe it. What was even more surprising was that milk, the usual food of choice in the treatment of stomach ulcers, was the one food that *did* inflame his stomach and aggravate the ulcer.

So do not be concerned about taking cayenne as a bitter herb. It will indeed improve your digestion, and it will not cause any problem, unless, as is the case with any food or substance, you are allergic to it.

Eating curry is probably the most pleasant way to take cayenne. Alternatively, you can get it as the herbal tincture. Remember that, as with all bitters, it will only do its job when you can taste it. It won't be helpful if you take it in a sealed capsule that does not break down until well in your digestive system. You want it to exert its action in your mouth.

- To make an infusion, put ¼ teaspoon in a cup of hot water and allow to infuse for ten minutes. Use one teaspoonful of this infusion, add hot water, and drink when needed.

Gentian Root

Gentian is an excellent sialogogue, but it is an even more useful bitters to help the stomach, as will be discussed under the stomach section. If you want to know more, now have a quick peek ahead (p.92).

Ginger

Ginger, which also goes under the lovely name of *Zingiber officinale*, is not only beneficial but tastes good. The root is the part that is used, and your best option is to add some of this fresh root to your cooking, as is done in India, China, and other parts of the world. Anytime you make a sauce, steam vegetables, stir-fry rice, or make a curry, you can incorporate grated fresh ginger root. However, you should avoid the ginger root that has been soaked in or coated with sugar; the sugar will be far from beneficial.

Ginger is an analgesic, antifungal, anti-inflammatory, antihistamine, carminative, diaphoretic, digestive stimulant, rubefacient, and general stimulant. That is a lot of activity, and clearly ginger has a lot to offer both in a Detox Regime and for your general health. As a diaphoretic, it will increase perspiration, and allow you to get rid of toxins through the skin.

Within the digestive system, it stimulates the flow of saliva, stimulates digestion generally, and so helps to relieve dyspepsia and flatulence. It has also been used in the treatment of colitis and diverticulitis. As an antifungal, it will help if you have problems with candida, particularly in the digestive tract.

As a further aid in Detox, ginger will give your immune system a good boost and help to prevent colds. Put slices of fresh ginger root in hot water for a refreshing and nose-clearing drink. As far as the rest of your health goes, ginger is very good for your heart, helping to prevent atherosclerosis, lower cholesterol levels, and prevent oxidation of the harmful low-density lipoproteins (LDLs), the ones that keep toxins circulating in your bloodstream, as well as stimulating the circulation and thus helping to prevent chilblains. This is also helpful if you suffer from arthritis or rheumatism, and ginger has been used externally in the treatment of fibrositis and muscle sprains.

Licorice Root

Licorice root has been suggested as a useful stimulant to get your digestive system off to a good start. However, its main action is on the colon, where it is helpful in the treatment of constipation. So again, if you want to know more, peek ahead (p.110).

Thyme

In spite of its name, *Thymus vulgaris*, one of the *Labiatae*, is not in the least vulgar. In fact, it is a delicate plant and offers many benefits as an herbal preparation. It is easy to grow, and if you have it in your garden or in pots, collect the leaves and flowers in summer while the plant is still flowering, usually in July and August. You may be surprised by how much this herb can do. Thyme acts as an antifungal, antimicrobial, antispasmodic, astringent, carminative, and expectorant, and improves circulation; the oil is an antioxidant.

While not often thought of as a medicinal herb, it is worth a mention here, since in addition to conferring so many benefits, it is so readily available in most kitchens and many herb gardens. All you need to do is add it to your cooking more often to provide extra flavor as well as health benefits.

It is useful in the treatment of many digestive problems. It will stimulate a sluggish digestive system and help in cases of dyspepsia, which can often be due to a simple lack of digestive activity. This in turn can lead to food just "sitting" in the stomach and then fermenting and producing unwanted gases. In addition, thyme can help further down the digestive tract, as it acts against molds such as *Candida albicans*, worms, and other parasites, and helps to eliminate them. As an antispasmodic, it can help in cases of spastic colon and irritable bowel syndrome.

This same action against unwanted parasites makes thyme a

useful herb to gargle with for sore throats, laryngitis, tonsillitis, and oral thrush, thus helping to clean up your mouth and throat. It is also useful in the treatment of respiratory infections such as ticklish coughs, whooping cough, bronchitis, and asthma. Again, use it as a gargle, and then swallow the liquid for the benefit it can also provide to the whole digestive system. It can be used in combination with sage for this purpose.

Thyme can also be used externally, and makes a useful antiseptic when applied to skin lesions.

- When making an infusion, allow two teaspoons of the dried herb to each cup of boiling water. If you prefer the tincture, the usual dose is ten drops to a teaspoon three times a day.

Refining Your Choice of Herbs

Let's sum up what has been considered so far. Gentian is generally considered one of the best herbs for getting your digestive system off to a good start, since it stimulates the flow of saliva and is also an excellent herb to use to improve stomach function. However, you might prefer to use cayenne if you have a stomach or duodenal ulcer, if you get frequent colds, or more prosaically and practically, if you enjoy curries. Similarly, you might choose ginger if you get colds and flu frequently and like its flavor, if you also have atherosclerosis or related cardiovascular problems, or if you are arthritic or suffer from rheumatism. Licorice, on the other hand, would be your choice if you also suffer from constipation, and again, of course, because you like the taste of it. If candidiasis is part of your problem then sialogogues that are also antifungal, such as ginger and thyme, are worth considering.

This is not only a specific comment about how to choose your sialogogue, but an example of the way you should go about choosing the most appropriate herb for you from each of the sections below. The method is the same, even though I won't be doing it for you each time. Make a note of the herbs you think will help you as you go along. There may be many occasions where the benefits overlap.

Herbs That Help Your Stomach

Probably the most important role of your stomach is to produce sufficient hydrochloric acid to trigger off an efficient digestive process. Without adequate production of acid here, there is a knock-on effect that affects your entire digestive system. Without the stimulus of hydrochloric acid from your stomach, your pancreas won't produce sufficient alkali or sufficient digestive enzymes for normal digestion within your small intestine. This in turn can lead to an environment that encourages pathogenic organisms, and all of this can then lead to constipation, and so on. This is so important we should say it again and again.

Fortunately, there are many herbs that can stimulate the stomach and help it to produce the necessary acids. They are known as *bitters*. Bitters do not, strictly speaking, just act on the stomach. They are, as their name implies, bitter or astringent to the taste, and they stimulate appetite and hence, rather like the action of increased saliva flow, stimulate the rest of your digestive system as well as your stomach.

There is one thing to be warned of with these herbs. Like sialogogues, there is little point in taking them in capsule or tablet form, such that you cannot taste them. It is the taste of the bitterness that stimulates the action. This action starts on your tongue and taste buds and goes from there via your brain to your digestive system, particularly the upper part, including your esophagus, stomach, liver, gallbladder, and pancreas.

Barberry

Barberry or *Berberis vulgaris*, is a bitter stomachic tonic, and as such, is a good herb for stimulating digestion and dealing with dyspepsia. However, it is also of great value to the liver, so you will need to look at p.131 for a more complete description.

Centaury

Technically known as *Erythraea centaurium* and part of the *Gentianaceae* family, centaury acts as a bitter, aromatic, mild nervine and gastric stimulant, so it is of obvious use in the digestive system.

It helps in conditions of sluggish digestion, dyspepsia, and poor liver function, particularly when combined with meadowsweet, marsh mallow root, and chamomile. It is also of use in cases of loss of appetite.

This is a good herb to choose if one of your additional problems involves stress or tension.

Gentian Root

Gentian root, or *Gentiana lutea,* to give it its Latin name, is one of the most frequently prescribed bitters. We mentioned it as a sialogogue, but it is now time to discuss it in greater detail. It is the rhizome and root of the herb that is used, and this should be dug up in autumn. In action, it is a bitter, gastric stimulant, sialagogue, cholagogue, choleretic, diuretic, anti-inflammatory, antibacterial, and stimulates the taste buds. What does all this mean? You will, of course, be checking back to the Herbal Functions table on p.57 to unravel these terms until you get used to them.

Within the digestive system, its main area of action, gentian has multiple uses and is often the herb of choice. It helps to stimulate a poor appetite. It stimulates and normalizes the production and flow of both saliva in the mouth and hydrochloric acid in the stomach, and this benefits digestion not only in the mouth and stomach, but has that knock-on benefit further down the digestive tract, as these fluids further stimulate the production of digestive enzymes from the pancreas and small intestine. Thus, gentian is an excellent herb to use if you have a sluggish digestive system. It is used in the treatment of dyspepsia, flatulence, and other symptoms of poor digestion. In addition, it is helpful in the treatment of a number of parasites including *Salmonella typhii* and *E. coli.*

It benefits the liver, containing components that are useful in the treatment of hepatitis; and as a choleretic, it stimulates the production and normal flow of bile, the net result of which is an improvement in or normalization of fat digestion and better bowel action.

As regards its actions that are peripheral to our discussion, as an anti-inflammatory and antibacterial agent it has been used in the treatment of malaria. It has also been used in the treatment of rheumatism.

- To make a decoction, allow ½ a teaspoon of the dried herb per cup. Alternatively, take betwen ¼ and 1 teaspoon of the tincture three times a day.

Golden Seal

Golden seal, or *Hydrastis canadensis,* from the *Ranunculaceae* or buttercup family is another herb with a multitude of uses. Its list of actions is impressive: anti-inflammatory, antipyretic, antifungal, anticatarrhal, antimalarial, antiparasitic, anodyne, astringent, laxative, muscular stimulant, bitter, oxytocic, and tonic. In addition to all that, it combines well with many other herbs. It will be discussed further when we consider the lymphatic system, for it has a great deal to offer there. For the moment, we are particularly interested in the digestive system, and here golden seal offers many benefits.

It is used in the treatment of many problems throughout the digestive tract, starting in the mouth, where it is used in the treatment of mouth ulcers and gum disease. If you have bleeding gums, a coated tongue or bad breath resulting from any infection or bacteria in the mouth, you can use this herb as a mouthwash. It is useful in the stomach to stimulate the production of stomach acid and in the treatment of gastritis and stomach ulcers. Remember that even when you have a stomach ulcer, you still need the normal production of stomach acid to promote healthy digestion. Use this herb and others to promote healing and remedies such as slippery elm powder to protect the damaged area in the meantime.

In the intestines, golden seal is used to treat duodenal ulcers, diverticulitis, colitis, Crohn's disease, and candidiasis. In all these situations, it is antiparasitic, helping to eradicate any toxic organisms that may be present and causing infections and local damage. As an anodyne it reduces the pain of ulcers and similar problems, and promotes healing. If you are concerned about having a leaky gut, then this is an important herb for you to consider.

As a laxative, it will help to prevent constipation, normalize bowel function, and reduce the formation of new toxins and the possibility of their absorption into your bloodstream. As a result of its astringent action it can help to stop bleeding, internally and externally; and a local application, usually as a cream, can help in the treatment of hemorrhoids. It also helps in some conditions of diarrhea.

When using it externally, it is good to remember that it is a strong dye and may stain clothing. It is not generally thought of as a particularly attractive plant and is rarely seen in gardens.

Wormwood

Wormwood, or *Artemisia absinthum,* from the *Compositae* family is an anthelmintic, anti-inflammatory, carminative, and bitter tonic and is useful when there is poor digestion and lack of sufficient stomach acid. As an anthelmintic, it is particularly useful when there are worms in the digestive tact, including roundworms and pinworms.

It has other uses too. Spread around, in combination with rue if you have it, it helps to repel fleas, moths, and other insects. It can be layered in drawers to protect clothing or strewn in your kitchen cupboards to reduce infections to foods.

- Make an infusion from 2 teaspoons of the leaves per cup, or take ½ to 1 teaspoonful three times a day.

What This Means for Your Stomach

It is time to summarize again. As far as your stomach is concerned, gentian is an excellent herb to help stimulate normal digestion, however, there are alternatives. For instance, if you also suffer from a sluggish liver and gallbladder, then you might prefer barberry; if you have stomach or duodenal ulcers, or an overgrowth of *Candida albicans,* then golden seal offers many other benefits; and if you have worms, wormwood would be a better choice. All of these herbs will help to stimulate the stomach and encourage its normal function within your digestive system.

Herbs for Flatulence

I nearly always ask patients if they burp or pass wind. The common reply is often, "Not really, only the usual amount." Yet it is debatable if you should produce gas or wind at all. Many people don't, and as people's health improves, it is common to find that they also stop producing wind.

In the long term, if you suffer from dyspepsia — the production of wind in the stomach — and a frequent need to burp to let out the unwanted gases, you should aim to improve your digestion as outlined here and prevent the problem from occurring at all. However, if burping and flatulence are a significant and uncomfortable part of your starting problem, you may want a short-term and immediate fix while you work on the long-term solutions to the problem, particularly if it is severe and immediate. Letting out the gas is not necessarily a part of a Detox Regime, but it may well be a part of the symptoms you are experiencing, particularly if part of your problem is the result of faulty digestion and toxins within the digestive tract.

Herbal treatments may take some time to produce a result, as herbs tend to bring about a slow and steady improvement, giving your body a chance to grow back to better health in its own natural way. This is in contrast to the sudden benefits you might expect from the more dramatic medical drugs. However, you should keep in mind that these medical drugs are overriding the function of your own body, forcing a change, at least for as long as you take them. They are not necessarily contributing to a long-term solution. They also tend to have unwanted and toxic side effects.

Take the case of antacids and other medical drugs used to relieve flatulence. They will work, or at least they will remove the immediate and obvious symptoms and will do so for as long as you take them, but you will probably have to carry them around with you at all times, to have them handy each time the problem occurs. They are doing nothing to stimulate your normal digestive processes. In addition, many of them contain sugar, not good for your health, and aluminium, which is definitely harmful.

Herbs, on the other hand, have the effect of stimulating the return of your organs to a normal and healthy function, with the result that you do not need to take them long-term. Any side effects they produce, at the normal therapeutic doses, are generally good ones, since most of them exert beneficial effects on more than one part of your body.

Let's get back to dyspepsia. We will assume that you have selected the combination of herbs you think you need for your overall detox plan insofar as it aims to improve your digestion. Now you are out at a restaurant, eating with friends or simply dining at home, and you are suddenly feeling bloated and uncomfortable. What can you do? There are a number of simple remedies that are probably close at hand to relieve the situation until your longer-term therapy produces the required result. They include such common herbs as peppermint, rosemary, celery, cumin, and coriander. In fact, it is common, in some cultures, to serve a small dish of these various seeds for people to nibble on at the end of a meal for just this purpose, as well as for their flavor.

If, after a meal, you feel bloated and full of wind, then consider having a cup of peppermint tea. This will help to relieve the situation. If you commonly suffer from flatulence, consider adding such seeds as celery, cumin, or cardamom to your meal itself. Dill seeds are also helpful. You may recall the old remedy of dill water for babies with colic. This works for the same reason, by making it easier for the baby to burp and release the gas.

If all else fails and you are desperate, take a charcoal tablet. Charcoal, whether as powder or as a tablet that breaks down in your gut, has a vast and highly absorbing surface area. It is able to absorb the gas and relieve your immediate symptoms, and to do so without other unwanted side effects. Remember, however, that this has not solved the problem long-term; you must still find the cause and correct it.

Peppermint

The leaves of *Mentha piperita* (*Labiatae*) are best collected just before the flowers open. Like all the mints, it grows rampant. It is easy to grow for yourself, but you would be well advised to keep it in a pot or in some area where its spread is contained. It is an aromatic, astringent, antispasmodic, anti-emetic, analgesic, carminative, and nervine.

It helps digestion and makes an excellent drink to have after a meal. It can be used to treat bloating and flatulence, relieve trapped wind, and cure dyspepsia. Use it in the treatment of headaches and migraines that are associated with indigestion.

Because of its relaxing and analgesic effect on the stomach

walls, it reduces the tendency to cause vomiting in pregnancy or during travel.

As a diaphoretic, it is an excellent remedy for colds and the flu, increasing the elimination of toxins via the skin, and the vapor helps to clear blocked sinuses and nasal passages and to relieve sinus headaches. Use it with boneset, elder, and yarrow for colds and the flu.

It should not be confused with spearmint, *Mentha spicata*, which is the herb usually used to make mint sauce. This is also an anti-spasmodic, carminative, stomachic, though less so than pepper-mint. It is also a mild diuretic.

There are countless other herbs for relieving flatulence. We have already mentioned the many spices that are useful. You will find others by looking down the column on table 1 (p.57) for carmi-natives.

ANTIFLATULENCE TEAS

Combine approximately equal amounts of peppermint leaves, chamomile flowers, and anise and caraway seeds. Add boiling water, allowing one to two teaspoons per cup, and leave to steep until cool enough to drink. One cup of this after a meal should help to solve the problem until such time as you no longer produce the unwanted gases.

If you prefer to do without the spices, combine equal amounts of chamomile, fennel, peppermint, and lemon balm leaves. Pour in boiling water, allowing for two teaspoons of the fresh herbs to each cup.

Herbs That Help Your Intestines

Small Intestine

Several types of digestive problems can occur in the small intes-tine, but they are usually resolved by dealing with other parts of your digestive tract. For instance, wind in the small intestine is a part of flatulence through your large and small intestine. Damage to the lining of your small intestine is dealt with by slippery elm and aloe vera juice, as it is for both stomach and colon problems. Poor digestion in the small intestine is generally resolved by the sialogogues and bitters that get good digestion started in your stomach and stimulate pancreatic function, and by herbs that improve the function of your liver and gallbladder.

Furthermore, it is generally difficult for you to distinguish between problems in the small and large intestines, since both lie within your lower abdomen. So we will deal with colon problems, and allow that anything you do there will almost certainly help both intestines.

Leaky Gut

A leaky gut, or gut permeability, is one local problem that you will want to attend to. This can be helped by a number of astringent herbs to stop bleeding; by demulcents to soothe; and by vulnerary herbs to promote healing. These same herbs can help in the treatment of colitis, mucous colitis, Crohn's disease, and other problems involving damaged lining of the intestinal tracts. All the herbs here are mentioned in more detail elsewhere in the book, in sections more specifically related to Detox, so only a brief mention is made of them in this section.

Useful *astringents* include bayberry, helpful in the treatment of leaky gut, diarrhea, dysentery, and mucous colitis; golden seal, an excellent herb for problems involving all the mucous membranes; and yellow dock, which also stimulates the liver, helps to prevent constipation, and is a blood cleanser. Culinary herbs that are astringent include caraway and cinnamon.

Helpful *demulcents* include aloe vera juice, an excellent demulcent; vulnerary, a valuable healing agent and promoter of new tissue repair; and bearberry, which has the additional benefit of being effective against a number of parasites. Marsh mallow, also an emollient and a vulnerary, is a particularly useful herb for mouth ulcers, stomach and duodenal ulcers, and healing the intestinal lining. Milk thistle is less specific for a leaky gut but would be the herb to choose if you also want to improve your liver function. Mullein is generally considered to be a demulcent specific to lung problems but can also be useful in the gut, particularly as it is also vulnerary. Licorice is excellent, as it is also an antiinflammatory and a mild laxative.

Slippery elm in powder form is one of the best remedies. A teaspoonful of this mashed into some food, such as a banana, and taken three times a day at eight-hour intervals will help to put an internal bandage along the lining of the gut. If you then drink aloe vera juice to act in its vulnerary role, you can heal most problems relating to damage to the intestinal tract lining. Fenugreek is a demulcent usually used for the lungs, but you could also include it in cooking.

Colon Problems

A number of malfunctions in your colon can lead to the buildup of toxins, which can then be absorbed through the walls of your colon and into your bloodstream, where they can do systemic damage throughout your body. It used to be believed that you only absorbed substances from your small intestine, not from the large one, but this is now considered to be wrong. In fact, the toxins absorbed from your colon can travel through your bloodstream and reach the kidneys, which then filter them out as they enter your urine.

Thus, it is important that your colon functions normally for two reasons. If it doesn't, you can both create more toxins there and, when you are constipated, hold on to the unwanted toxins you should be expelling.

What happens in your colon? Undigested food leaves your small intestine in a liquid mush. Ideally this undigested food should be the nondigestible carbohydrates you have eaten, commonly and erroneously referred to as "fiber." Unfortunately, if your digestive system is inefficient, it may also contain foods that would otherwise have been broken down and absorbed, such as undigested fats or protein. In addition, it contains microorganisms, dead or alive, and of course, a lot of water. Many of the microorganisms are beneficial, but if the conditions are not as they should be, they may favor the presence of a variety of unwanted and harmful organisms.

How Often Should You Go?

A necessary part of any Detox Regime is proper elimination from your bowels. If you are constipated, then toxins can develop, accumulate, and be absorbed into your bloodstream from where they are carried throughout your body. You will be creating the problem, not solving it.

How often should you go? We have already touched on this, but it is definitely worth repeating, and besides, you may just have dipped into this book here. Most people feel they are doing well if they have one bowel motion a day and do not worry if they skip a day or two each week. But think about it. If you eat three meals a day, surely you should "go" three times a day. If you do not, then obviously some waste material is sitting there, waiting for the next exit, and during this time it can do harm.

Not only is this concept theoretically plausible, but studies have shown that in communities where there is a high fiber intake from a diet rich in vegetables, fruit, and whole grains, most people do indeed go several times a day; and they produce large, soft movements that are easily passed. Not only that, but they have only a fraction, often as little as 5 percent, of the bowel problems common in our society, including diverticulitis, colon cancer, and hemorrhoids.

So, if you are not "going" three times a day, what do you have to do to correct the situation?

Bulking agents Normal colon function is maintained by the peristaltic action of the muscle walls of your colon as they progressively sweep the contents along. This peristalsis is stimulated by the presence of bile acids and bile salts from your gallbladder and by the pressure of the bulk of the stool on the walls of your colon. As the stool moves along at the correct speed, an appropriate amount of water is drawn from it and reabsorbed back through the colon walls into your bloodstream. If this did not happen, you would have a very liquid stool indeed and soon become severely dehydrated.

If peristalsis is limited, as a result of insufficient bulk, inadequate production of bile, or due to some other cause, then too much fluid is reabsorbed, the stool becomes hard and small, and transit along the colon becomes progressively more slow and more difficult. Constipation, and the accompanying production and absorption of toxins, are the obvious results.

A word about fiber If you are constipated and plan to improve the situation, you will almost certainly think about one or both of two possible solutions to the problem: increasing the fiber content of your diet or taking laxatives.

We'll start with fiber. What is it? The word *fiber* is actually a misnomer. Many of the things that act to increase the bulk of the stool are not actually fibrous. Using the term fiber leads to images of scratchy brooms scrubbing out the walls of the colon. As a result, many people with abdominal pain or pain that they associate with their colon are reluctant to increase their fiber intake.

A better term for such substances, even though it is a mouthful, is "nondigestible carbohydrates." These nondigestible carbohydrates possess a number of attributes and do a number of things. First, because, by definition, you cannot digest them yourself, you cannot absorb them into your system. As a result, they go on through your small intestine relatively intact and enter your colon. Here they provide valuable food for the microorganisms of your lower digestive tract. After all, if you could digest and absorb 100 percent of the food you ate, what would these organisms in your colon have to live on? So, these organisms then consume part of these nondigestible carbohydrates, and as a result they increase in number and make up a significant part (up to 50 percent) of the dry weight of your stool.

Second, most of these nondigestible carbohydrates have the capacity to absorb and hold water. This means that instead of the stool drying out and becoming too hard and difficult to pass, it remains relatively wet, bulky, and soft. This soft material is then easier to pass, just because it is soft. In addition to that, because of the increased bulk, it puts gentle pressure on the walls of the colon and this then stimulates these walls into further and appropriate action. The peristaltic action that results is a wavelike motion that propels the waste material along your colon, toward the exit.

Third, simply by being there, these carbohydrates themselves contribute to the bulk of the waste material and therefore enhance this effect.

So what should you do? Clearly you should increase the amount of fiber in your diet; you should increase the amount of nondigestible carbohydrate. The question is, how?

Fiber, as we have seen, may or may not be fibrous. In the obvious examples of many vegetables, clearly it *is* fibrous. However, the nondigestible carbohydrates in linseeds, slippery elm powder, and psyllium hulls are not fibrous. In whatever form it comes, it *must* survive the digestive tract so it can provide food for the colon bacteria and absorb water to increase the bulk of the stool, and you must have plenty of it.

There are several ways to achieve this outcome. The first thing to consider is your intake of vegetables and, to a lesser extent, fruit. Here, much of the nondigestible carbohydrate is indeed fibrous, as the strings on celery or those along the pods of green beans show all too clearly. However, it is still true that not all the nondigestible carbohydrates of vegetables are actually fibrous.

Ideally, your diet should contain a large amount of vegetables. I choose my words carefully. Most patients tell me they do indeed eat "a lot of vegetables," yet in practice this may not be the case. I recall one patient whose only vegetable, eaten at every meal, was a single serving of frozen peas. I told her she should eat more vegetables. On her next visit, she proudly informed me that she now ate sixteen vegetables every single day. I was pleased for her until I discovered she had made a vegetable stew of sixteen different vegetables, frozen the mixture, and then served up a single spoonful of this for her dinner each evening.

Many patients tell me they eat lots of vegetables, but this may only mean that they have perhaps two or three for dinner. They almost certainly have none for breakfast, and probably very little fruit either, and they generally have very few or only a small amount at lunchtime.

Measure this against a Stone Age diet, thought to have consisted of about 80 percent fruit and vegetables, and you will see that there is a large discrepancy. Given the social habits of today, you may not achieve this intake level, but if you are not having three soft and easy bowel motions every day, our definition here of avoiding constipation, then do try to include at least some fruit or vegetable at every meal, and increase the quantities progressively.

Vegetable and fruit fiber is much better for you than cereal fiber, so taking extra spoonfuls of bran is not the answer. Some people are allergic to the grains, often without knowing it. Other people may find that large amounts of bran actually slow down the digestive processes unless they drink a lot of water at the same time. If you are going to eat cereal fiber, the bran from the different grains, it is best eaten as part of the whole grain. It is better to always eat wholemeal flour rather than sometimes eating white flour and then compensating with a tablespoon of bran. Eat brown rice rather than the low-fiber white rice. Eat oat cakes or rye-based biscuits rather than ones made of wheat (one of the most common allergens, and all too often refined of its fiber).

The second way to solve problems of constipation and ensure proper peristalsis is to provide sufficient bulk from other, non-food sources such that the pressure of the colon contents on the walls of the colon acts as the trigger to increased movement. This peristalsis should be achieved, if possible, by the vegetable and fruit fiber as discussed above. However, years of a low-fiber diet can lead to a very sluggish system, and you may need extra help to get it going again.

This extra bulk can be added to your daily intake by including a number of substances such as slippery elm powder, ground psyllium hulls, or linseeds, whole or ground. These are discussed in full later on.

Whatever forms of nondigestible carbohydrate you choose, there is another important ingredient that you need to achieve the solution you are after. That is water. If all the fiber in your diet comes from fruits and vegetables, they themselves will provide most of the water needed. However, if you do not drink sufficient water each day, then you will not have sufficient bulk. Instead, the fiber may just "sit" there and gum the works up even further.

Ideally, of course, this liquid should be drunk sometime removed from actually eating your meal. You need to have concentrated digestive juices to work on the food you have eaten. So make a practice of drinking plenty of fluids throughout the day. If you forget, then have a drink a short while before eating. Don't use liquid to try to flush your food down a reluctant digestive tract.

Having said that, there is evidence that will make the dedicated wine imbiber happy. It seems that one glass of wine with a meal may actually help to stimulate the flow of digestive juice, acting as a bitters. You might conceivably stretch this to a second glass, particularly if it is a red wine or a particularly dry white wine, but no more. After that, you are almost certainly doing more harm than good as you increase the work of your liver in breaking down the alcohol. I suggest, however, that this is not a reason to start drinking if you do not already do so. Use bitter herbs instead to achieve the same outcome, and eat fresh fruits and red grapes to get the antioxidants found in red wine. But if you are going to drink anyway, then holding it to this level and type can help to soothe your conscience. Furthermore, having a glass of wine generally means that you are going to eat more slowly and be more relaxed as you eat, and this in itself is a benefit to your digestive system.

It's now time to consider some examples of useful and nutritious nondigestible carbohydrates that are not part of a person's normal diet.

Linseeds

Linseeds, *Linum usitatissimum* from the *Linaceae* family — also called flaxseeds — are small, flat, and shiny brown seeds. They are emollient, demulcent, and pectoral. The nondigestible carbohydrate in linseed is not fibrous, but it does absorb water and does swell up in the colon. To see what this means, put a tablespoon of linseeds in a glass of warm water at about body heat and watch what happens. You will see the whole thing set into a type of soft jelly. This is just the beneficial action that happens inside your digestive tract.

The other important ingredients of linseeds are the highly unsaturated fatty acids.

Linseeds can be eaten either ground or whole. However, since they contain highly unsaturated fats that can easily be oxidized and go rancid, it is better to eat them whole. If you do choose to grind them, then grind them freshly each time you eat some. If you are eating them primarily for their bulking action, it does not matter if you swallow them whole or chew them. If you wish to benefit from some of their essential fatty acid content, then it is important that you chew them or grind them. You can grind them in a small coffee bean grinder or something equivalent.

- How much is enough? The simple answer is "Enough to get you going." You could start by taking a tablespoon two or three times a day. Make sure you drink a large glass of water or other similar liquid with it.

Psyllium Hulls

The seeds of psyllium or *Plantago psyllium* from the *Plantaginaceae* family are usually available in ground form. Sometimes they are referred to as psyllium hulls. They contain nondigestible carbohydrates that absorb water and so hold it in the stool. Psyllium is a gentle laxative, demulcent, and emollient.

Psyllium hulls have another benefit. The soluble fiber portion absorbs a variety of toxins as it passes through your gut. These toxins may be chemical toxins of all sorts, such as those added to your foods in the various growing and processing stages. They also include internally produced toxins such as those produced by the mold *Candida albicans*. By absorbing these toxins onto the psyllium hulls, you can reduce the amount you yourself absorb into your bloodstream, and so can reduce the symptoms the toxins and organisms cause. Further, when you are actively treating candidiasis, there is generally an increased release of these chemicals into your digestive tract, leading to a temporary but unpleasant increase in your own symptoms. This effect is often referred to as the "die-off effect." It can be reduced significantly if you eat psyllium hulls at the same time. These hulls may also help you to eliminate the organism itself and to absorb and eliminate the bodies of other parasites, dead or alive. If you lust for desserts but are trying to resist the following is a solution provided by one of my patients.

Paulene was both seriously constipated and seriously overweight. Each day she allowed herself one glass of fresh fruit juice. She added her ground psyllium hulls to this and allowed it to set like a jelly. Eating it took a lot longer than drinking the juice would have done and allowed her to have both her dessert and a clean conscience.

Slippery Elm Powder

The name says it all. This is a powder made from the inner bark of the elm tree, *Ulmus fulva*, and when it is mixed with water, it is indeed slippery or mucilaginous. It is collected in early spring and offers many advantages, particularly, but not exclusively, to your digestive system. We have already seen how it can help a leaky gut.

It is astringent, a gentle-acting demulcent, an emollient, and a nutrient. The mucilaginous substances in it combine with the fluids in the digestive tract and cover the mucous membranes with a protective layer. This is somewhat analogous to putting an internal bandage along the walls of your digestive system. It can cover areas of ulceration or abrasion, as well as areas that have been damaged by molds and fungi such as *Candida albicans* or by other organisms. It can cover areas that have been damaged when you have been bloated and the colon walls have been distended abnormally. And there is more: the mucilage then stimulates normal mucosal secretion, and this in turn helps to improve and normalize your digestive function.

This means that slippery elm powder is useful in cases of esophagitis, where the esophagus is inflamed or painful, a condition sometimes referred to as heartburn. It can reduce the pain felt when you have a hiatal hernia, although it will not actually alter the presence of the hernia itself. Use slippery elm powder when there is inflammation of the stomach lining, as in gastritis, or where there are stomach or duodenal ulcers. People suffering from Crohn's disease, intestinal thrush, an inflamed small intestine (ileitis), an inflamed colon (colitis), or diverticulitis (inflamed pockets in the colon wall) will benefit from the use of slippery elm powder.

In addition to all that, it will help directly in our Detox Regime. Like the other two bulking agents, linseeds and psyllium hulls, by holding water in the stool, it increases the bulk of the stool and thus helps to prevent constipation.

Slippery elm powder was drunk by previous generations as a nutritious evening drink, maybe in much the same way that we now drink Ovaltine or hot chocolate. It was mixed well with milk; the mixture brought to a boil; allowed to simmer for ten minutes; then flavored with cinnamon, mace, or nutmeg and sweetened with honey. Try it for yourself as a pleasant way to drink it. You will have to take care when getting it to mix with the milk or it can become lumpy.

Another way to take it, one that most of my patients find to be easier than trying to make a drink of it, is to mix it with half a banana mashed thoroughly. The mashed banana is itself mucilaginous or, not to put too fine a point on it, "slimy," and it largely hides the taste and texture of the slippery elm powder. One or two teaspoons of the powder two or three times a day (ideally at eight-hour intervals) will generally be sufficient for any abrasions or pain.

Combine the slippery elm powder with drinks of aloe vera juice to promote healing and you can improve the state of your digestive system enormously. To increase bowel motions and the general elimination of toxins, it is a good idea to combine it with psyllium hulls, linseed, or other insoluble fibers.

As a further benefit, slippery elm powder can also be made, with warm water, into a poultice for putting on abscesses, boils, and ulcers.

A word of warning. Be careful what you buy. There are products available called Slippery Elm Food; they even claim to be 100 percent pure slippery elm food. This may lull you into thinking that pure slippery elm powder is exactly what you are getting, with nothing else added. In practice, some of them contain as little as 2 percent slippery elm powder, the other 98 percent being made up of flour, milk powder, sugar, and other ingredients that are of no particular benefit. Ask for absolutely 100 percent pure slippery elm.

If you cannot get slippery elm in powder form, then the capsules will do if you are trying to prevent constipation. However, they are not good if you want to protect your esophagus or upper stomach, as it takes the capsules some time to break down after you have swallowed them. By the time that they *do* open up, they may have passed the place where their action is required.

Again, you may be wondering how much. The answer is, whatever is sufficient to get you going. Remember that this is also a nutritive and was once used as a drink, so you can have as much as you want or need, provided, of course, that you drink plenty of fluid with it.

Action of Bulking Agents

These three bulking agents, in addition to holding water in the stool, will themselves contribute to the bulk of the stool, make it larger and softer, and help to prevent constipation. They will help to eliminate toxins that are present and to reduce the formation of new and putrefactive toxins.

Although it may sound strange at first, these bulking agents can also be used in the opposite situation, when there is diarrhea, for exactly the same reason and by the same mechanism. They will "hold" the liquid in the loose motion that is flowing too rapidly, thus setting it and firming it up. As a result of this, the transit speed is reduced, normal reabsorption of water across the colon walls and back into your system can take place, and the diarrhea can be halted.

A further benefit of these actions will be felt if you have hemorrhoids. By making the stool softer and easier to pass, there will be less pressure on the tissues around the exit and less straining. This means that there is less of a tendency to create hemorrhoids and that any hemorrhoids present have a better chance to heal.

Aperients, Laxatives, and Cathartics

There are other ways to get your bowels working, although they are generally not as good as bulking agents, at least from the point of view of your long-term health — although they may get good results initially. This is the use of the groups of herbs that are aperients, laxatives, cathartics, and purgatives. You will recall from the Herbal Functions table that aperients are very mild laxatives, whereas true laxatives are substances that have a strong stimulating effect on the bowel. Cathartics and purgatives are the strongest, and ensure rapid evacuation of the bowel contents.

Aperients, such as rhubarb, dandelion, and milk thistle, generally achieve their outcome by stimulating the flow of bile from your liver and gallbladder. This bile, in turn, acts on the walls of your colon and stimulates their peristaltic action, the wavelike motion that propels food along your digestive tract, particularly, in this case, the lower digestive tract. This is a gentle, effective, and appropriate way of stimulating normal elimination of waste products and has the added benefit of various positive actions on your liver and gallbladder themselves.

We will start with the aperients, then move on to stronger stuff. The most obvious herbs to think of, ranging from aperients to purgatives, are probably rhubarb root, licorice, dandelion, milk thistle, senna, and cascara sagrada. However, you will find that there are many other herbs with an action on the colon. I have selected quite a few, all with other beneficial actions as well, so that you can choose the one or ones that best suit your combination of symptoms or needs.

Bogbean

The leaves of bogbean, buckbean, or *Menyanthes trifoliata* from the *Menyanthaceae* family are bitter, diuretic, cholagogue, aperient, and antirheumatic. As a bitters, bogbean helps to stimulate digestion in the stomach; as a chologogue, it stimulates the flow of bile. The net effect is that of a gentle aperient that stimulates the colon. Bogbean should not be used if you suffer from diarrhea or have blood in your stools.

Elder

When is an herb not an herb? Elder is indeed a most useful herb, yet like some other so-called herbs, including the elm we have just been discussing, it is also a tree, both in its own right and with the help of any nearby tree through which it will climb and entwine.

Elder, or *Sambucus nigra*, a *Caprifoliaceae*, is usually thought of as an herb that helps to fight infections, particularly those due to viruses such as the common cold and influenza, and that indeed is what it does best

However, the berries, as any enthusiastic consumer of homemade elderberry wine will know, are a mild aperient, the flowers are laxative, the leaves are purgative, and the bark is purgative and emetic, so you can take your choice. Obviously it would be an herb to choose if you suffer from frequent viral infections or have a poor immune system as well, as needing help with respect to constipation.

It is available in various forms in most health-food stores, and this could also be a good excuse for you to sample some of the elderberry wines you can occasionally find.

Golden Seal

Golden seal has already been mentioned in detail when we discussed the stomach (p.93). Take another look at that section. For our purposes here, it is a gentle laxative that also has a healing effect on the digestive tact, which is obviously beneficial in any case of other digestive disturbance as well as constipation.

Licorice

Licorice is another herb, like ginger, that is often available in sweetened forms. However, any sugar that is added to the confectionary form is obviously not good for you, so choose the unsweetened form. There is also doubt as to just how much pure licorice there is in some of the confectionary products anyway, so again, they are best avoided.

Licorice, or *Glycyrrhiza glabra*, is part of the *Leguminosae* or bean family. The herbal preparation is made from the dried root of the plant, which is, in its natural form, slightly sweet and should not be harvested until the fourth year of growth.

The use of licorice as a medicinal herb has a long history going back to the time of the ancient Greeks, who used it as a pectoral in the treatment of coughs and asthma. The Romans knew of it, it was used in Germany in the Middle Ages, and in England in Elizabethan times.

Licorice is an anti-inflammatory, antispasmodic, demulcent, diuretic, expectorant, a mild laxative, and an adrenal agent, and clearly has many benefits throughout the body.

Within the digestive system, it is useful in the treatment of nausea, as a demulcent; anti-inflammatory and antispasmodic in the treatment of stomach ulcers, gastritis, abdominal pain, colic, colitis, and diverticulitis; and as a mild laxative in the treatment of constipation. It can also be used to hide the flavor of some of the less pleasant herbal tinctures.

Licorice has more to offer. It benefits the immune system, as we shall see later on. It benefits your adrenal glands, which are called into play whenever adrenalin is needed, such as when you are stressed or when your blood sugar level falls. It also helps to balance estrogen levels and reduce the symptoms of menopause. Licorice can help in all these situations, so if any of them apply to you *and* you are constipated, then this could be an excellent herb to choose.

As well as coming as a confectionary, licorice is available in salty form. This should, however, be avoided if you have high blood pressure.

- Add ½ to 1 teaspoon of the root to a cup of water, simmer for 15 minutes, and drink this three times a day. If you prefer, take the herbal tincture, ¼ teaspoon three times a day.

Dandelion

Dandelion, or *Taraxacum officinale* from the *Turneraceae* family, may be a common weed to many a gardener, but it is a wonderful herb for your liver and digestive system. It is a hepatic, chola-gogue, antirheumatic, laxative, and tonic. You can use the leaves as a diuretic, what's more, one that provides its own potassium, but we will focus for the moment on the root. This is not only an excellent herb for the liver, but it gently and successfully stimulates normal peristaltic action and prevents constipation, thus aiding the elimination of toxins in the intestines and reducing the chance of the formation of new ones.

You can buy dandelion coffee in almost any health-food store. Don't be put off by the word *coffee*. It is used simply to distinguish it, a drink based on the plant's root, from herb "teas" that use the leaves of the various herbs. You an also make dandelion coffee yourself (see p.127)

Milk Thistle

Milk thistle, *Silybum marianum* from the *Compositae* family, is another excellent herb that should be part of any Detox Regime. Like dandelion, it is mainly thought of as a liver herb, and it is discussed in detail in that section. But we also need to mention it briefly here because it is an excellent herb to get your bowels moving properly. Like dandelion and many other herbs mentioned here, it does this via its effect on the liver and by stimulating the normal flow of bile.

Wahoo

The root bark of Wahoo or *Euonymus atropurpureus* from the *Celastraceae* family is also known by the delightful name of spindle tree. It is a smooth-leaved shrub with purple flowers and purple edges to the leaves, found in hedgerows and woodlands. The root bark is a cholagogue, laxative, diuretic, and circulatory stimulant. Its greatest use is for liver problems including jaundice, for the treatment of gallstones, and gallbladder inflammation or pain. We will be discussing it in more detail later on.

However, it deserves a mention here because, as a result of its action on the liver and gallbladder, it is an excellent herb for mild constipation and helps to encourage good bowel movements.

Fringetree

Here we have another tree used in herbal medicine. The root bark of this tree, *Chionanthus virginicus*, is a cholagogue, hepatic, alterative, diuretic, tonic, and laxative.

It thus combines several actions that will help in any Detox Regime. As an alterative, it is a general cleanser and will help clean the blood and all the tissues. As a diuretic, it will help to eliminate unwanted fluid; and as a laxative, it will stimulate peristaltic action and clean out the colon. It is particularly useful if you have problems of fluid retention or problems with your liver and gallbladder, and is useful in cases of gallstones. We will be discussing this herb in the next chapter (p.134).

Rhubarb Root

Before you get excited and think this is an herb or plant you know well, be warned. Rhubarb root, also known as turkey rhubarb, East Indian rhubarb, or Russian rhubarb — the names all indicating the route it traveled to get from China to the West — is *Rheum palmatum* of the *Polygonaceae* family. It is not the common garden rhubarb found in many vegetable plots and turned into a dessert by the addition of a generous spread of sugar. But come to mention it, if you do grow this rhubarb and want to maintain a low level of sugar intake, then another herb by the name of sweet cicely should be grown nearby. When the two are cooked together, you need a lot less sugar to eliminate the bitter flavors in rhubarb. This is thought to be due, not to the fact that sweet cicely tastes sweet — it doesn't — but to the possible action it has in blocking the taste buds that pick up the sour and acid flavors in the rhubarb.

But back to turkey rhubarb or rhubarb root. It is a bitter, stomachic, laxative, mild purgative, and astringent. As this would suggest, it is useful in the treatment of both constipation and sluggish digestion. We are moving now from the gentle aperients to a more active laxative, so be careful with the amount you take and increase this slowly as you discover the effect it has on you. If you are using a decoction, start with ¼ teaspoon of the dried herb per cup, increasing gradually to twice this amount. Similarly with the tincture: start with one ml three times a day, increasing, if necessary, to double this amount. If it causes cramps, take it with a carminative such as aniseed, caraway, cardamom, chamomile, dill, ginger, or peppermint. Be warned, it may color your urine yellow or red. This is no cause for concern and does not suggest the presence of blood.

Cascara Sagrada

With Cascara sagrada or *Rhamnus purshiana* of the *Rhamnaceae* family, we move to even stronger herbs. The dried bark is used, in quill or powdered form, or it can be obtained as a tincture. It is a bitter, tonic, and laxative, and for this latter purpose it is effective but should be taken with care. Initially you should try some of the above herbs in conjuction with an improved diet. Only if the situation persists should you resort to cascara or senna.

Cascara is used in the treatment of habitual and persistent constipation. It acts directly to stimulate — some might even say irritate — the walls of the colon, by gently stimulating the flow of bile from the liver and gallbladder. It should only be used in acute situations and is not an appropriate long-term solution. It

may cause cramps, and if this occurs, you should use a carminative such as aniseed, peppermint, or ginger with it, but you might
be better advised to find an alternative treatment.

It is wise to combine this herb with some of the others discussed
above, such as licorice, dandelion, or milk thistle, as well as the
aromatic or carminative herbs to minimize cramping.

- To make a decoction, use one to two teaspoons of the dried
  herb per cup. If you are taking the tincture, start slowly and
  work up to a dose of ¼ teaspoon. Cascara should be taken last
  thing at night, and it generally acts by the morning.

Senna

There are two types of senna, *Cassia angustifolia* and *Cassia senna*,
and both are cathartic. Like cascara, senna should only be used
for short periods and in severe conditions of constipation. It too
may cause cramps and should be combined with carminative and
antispasmodics such as peppermint or chamomile, and with other
milder laxatives that work via the liver. As with cascara, you should
start out by taking only a small amount and tailor the dose until
you get the desired result. Do not plan to rely on its use. Instead,
you should do all you can to improve your diet and increase its
fiber content, use bulking agents such as linseed, and herbs to
improve your liver function.

What about Dates, Prunes, and Figs?

I can almost hear the question being asked. What about dried fruits
such as dates and figs? Surely they are laxative. The short answer
is no. Of themselves they are not laxative. Think about it. What
is a prune but a dried plum. You may claim that two or three
prunes keep you regular. Would three plums do the same? Almost
certainly not. What's the difference? It can hardly be the loss of
water that makes the prune more laxative than the plum since
you have already been advised to *increase* your intake of water to
help prevent constipation and to improve your Detox Regime. It's
the same with dates or figs — the organically grown fresh fruit
is not laxative; the commercially available dried fruits are.

The truth is, it is the pesticides that are used to fumigate the fruits when they are dried for the purpose of improving their shelf life that produce the laxative action. In effect, you are relying on the fumigants to irritate your colon sufficiently to stimulate its action and deal with the constipation. This is not a good plan.

Many of the dried fruit bars, promoted for the treatment of constipation, also contain senna or cascara, so remind yourself about the reservations regarding these herbs mentioned above.

A ONE-TIME CLEANOUT

If you are seriously constipated and need a good cleanout, try this combination:

Anise seed	1 part
Fennel seed	1 part
Milk thistle	5 parts
Dandelion root	5 parts
Licorice root	5 parts
Psyllium hulls	5 parts
Rhubarb root	5 parts
Senna	3 parts

If you can get the herbs in dry, powdered form, then make up the mixture and take a half a teaspoonful as a single dose. If this is insufficient, increase the dose until you get the desired effect. You can also make it into a decoction by simmering it in water for 15 minutes, allow 1 teaspoon to the cup, and start with half a cup. If you get the herbs as tinctures, then exclude dandelion, which you can drink as the coffee, and psyllium hulls, which you can take as prescribed on p.105. Combine the remaining tinctures, and take one teaspoonful initially, working up until you get the required action.

Remember that this contains senna, an intestinal irritant, and should not be used long-term. If you do want to use it over an extended period, leave out the senna after the initial cleanout.

Diverticulitis

There is another problem we should consider before leaving the colon. That is diverticulitis. Diverticulae are small blind pouches that form in the wall and lining of the colon. They may be caused by constipation where pressure on the walls of the colon leads to the formation of the pouches. They may also occur when there is weakness of the muscle walls of the colon. Once formed, they are small blind pockets that can easily become filled with waste material. When this ferments, bacteria and toxins can accumulate, the diverticulae then become inflamed, hence diverticulitis. In time they will cause pain, possibly due to trapped gases and associated with spasms and cramping.

The treatment should aim at removing the toxic material and consist of the use of mild aperients, such gentle bulking agents as slippery elm powder, and healers such as aloe vera. Gentle enemas have also been found to be helpful. Wild yam is a beneficial herb.

Wild Yam

Wild yam, or *Dioscorea villosa* from the *Dioscoreaceae* family and also known by the informative name of colic root, is a tropical plant most commonly grown in Africa and not one you are likely to find in a cool-climate herb garden. There are many different varieties of yam, and some may be familiar to you as a delicious form of sweet potato.

Dioscorea villosa is not so tasty; in fact, it is slightly bitter and has relatively little other taste. The woody roots are harvested in autumn, and dried to make the herbal remedy. It contains steroidal saponins such as dioscine; phytosterols such as diosgenin; (precursors to DHEA); alkaloids; tannin; and starch; and acts as an antispasmodic, anti-bacterial, anti-inflammatory, antirheumatic, and cholagogue.

This gives it several beneficial uses in the digestive system, and it is also helpful for gallbladder problems. As an antispasmodic, it has been used in the treatment of colic — with and without nausea — spastic colon, and irritable bowel syndrome. It is also helpful in the treatment of diverticulitis; in fact, it is probably one of the best herbs for this condition. For this purpose you should consider combining it with such gentle and relaxing herbs as chamomile and possibly a soft demulcent such as marsh mallow.

In addition, this would be a good herb to choose if you are going through menopause as it is said that it helps to balance the female hormones. It can also be used, earlier in life, to reduce the nausea of pregnancy, the cramps of the menstrual cycle, and ovarian and uterine pains. Still acting as an antispasmodic, it is helpful in the treatment of hiccups and asthma.

It is claimed to have a further benefit, and you may know what it is. It is thought to act on the endocrine or hormone system and lead to an increase in the body's level of progesterone. This is thought to be another reason why it is helpful in the treatment of dysmennorrhea and why it has been used by women going through menopause who do not want to take HRT. It is worth mentioning briefly that although there are negative concerns about taking HRT, there are also some concerns about taking progesterone on an extended basis, and these could extend to concerns over the long-term use of wild yam. However, that is part of a different story, one that we are not considering here.

Worms and Other Parasites

One of the tests I commonly do for patients — particularly but not exclusively those suffering from digestive upsets — is to test a stool sample for parasites — for a range of unwanted organisms such as molds, bacteria, and worms. It is surprising how often they are present and are part of the problem. If you feel you have any digestive problems, it may be worth investigating this. There is a very simple diagnostic test that can be easily organized by any naturopath or interested practitioner.

Part of any Detox Regime should involve making sure that you have no unwanted parasites in your gut. There are many herbs that can help to eradicate these unwanted visitors, and they can readily be incorporated into your Detox Regime.

If your digestion is perfect, then you may not need them, although going on my own clinical experience, you still may. If you are having problems with your digestive system, you would be very wise to include one or more of the herbs listed below.

For serious infestations, it is wise to follow the treatment indicated below with a dose of a cathartic such as cascara or senna to ensure maximum expulsion of the parasites.

Aloe

Aloe vera is discussed in more detail in the chapter on the skin. However, it is also an anthelmintic and will help to expel worms. It provides the added benefit of being healing, thereby helping to repair any damage the worms may have caused during their stay.

Black Walnut

The unripe hulls of *Juglans niger* (*Juglandaceae*) are antifungal, anthelminthic, antiviral, and antibacterial. The herb is used, in tincture form, in the treatment of infestations of many parasites including *Candida albicans*, *Salmonells sp.*, and pathogenic E.coli.

- For a decoction, allow 1 teaspoonful per cup; if using the tincture, take ¼ teaspoon three times a day.

Butternut

Related to black walnut, butternut, or *Juglans cinerea*, is anthelmintic, cathartic, tonic, and can be used to treat worms.

- Half to one teaspoon of the tincture should be taken three times a day.

Garlic

Garlic is discussed elsewhere (p.143) and is not generally described as an anthelmintic. However, it is not liked by worms or mold and, together with leeks and onions, if eaten in any quantity before a treatment does ensure a more successful outcome. It is effective against molds, particularly *Candida albicans*. For cases of athlete's foot, the result of a mold between the toes, a dusting with garlic powder will often get rid of the problem — if not some of your friends.

CUCUMBER WITH GARLIC AND YOGURT

This is another way to serve raw garlic and is an excellent dish to have with hot curry.

Peel and chop one cucumber. Crush three or four cloves of fresh garlic, combine with the cucumber, and place in a bowl. Add sufficient natural yogurt to cover the cucumber. Mix and serve decorated with mint leaves.

Pumpkin Seeds

The seeds of pumpkin, *Cucurbita pepo* (a cucurbitaceae), are harvested in the autumn when the fruit is ripe. They are anthelmintic and very useful in the treatment of worms and similar digestive system parasites. The seeds can be eaten and should be chewed thoroughly.

Quassia

The stem wood, without its bark, of *Picrasma excelsor* (a simarubaceae) is used. It is an anthelmintic, bitter, sialogogue, and tonic, so it can contribute in several ways to a Detox Regime.

As a sialogogue and bitter, it will stimulate your digestive system; as an anthelmintic, it will help to clear out worms and parasites; and as a tonic, it will give you an energy boost and tone up your whole system. It is particularly effective against threadworms. Externally it can be used for the treatment of lice.

• Take ¼ teaspoon of the tincture three times a day.

Tansy

The leaves of tansy, or *Tanacetum vulgare* (a compositae), are collected in summer. It is anthelmintic, bitter, carminative, emmenagogue, stimulant, tonic, and vermifuge.

Its main use is against worms, especially roundworm and threadworm. It can also be used externally as a wash for scabies and other parasites. If the leaves are strewn on kitchen shelves, they will help to keep ants and other insects away.

This herb is a strong emenogogue and should not be taken if you are pregnant.

- Make an infusion, allowing for a teaspoonful of the dried herb per cup, or take ¼ teaspoon of the tincture three times a day.

Thyme

Thyme is discussed elsewhere. It is useful anthelmintic and antiparasitic and is also effective against molds.

Wormwood

Wormwood was discussed in the section on the stomach. It is also one of the most useful anthelmintics, as it not only helps to expel parasites but also tones up the whole digestive system.

Marigold

Marigold is discussed in the chapter on the skin. It is worth a mention here, as it is a useful antifungal.

Olive Leaf

The leaves of olive, *Oleo europaea*, have many uses. The herb is antibacterial, antifungal, antimicrobial, antiviral; antioxidant, antiarrhythmic, hypoglycaemic, hypolipidemic, hypouricemic, hypocholesterolemic, and hypotensive. With a list of actions like this, it is not surprising to find that it acts on many different parts of the body.

It qualifies here, as it is effective against several different organisms including *Staphylococcus aureus*, E coli, and some molds. As an antibacterial, antiviral, antifungal, and general antimicrobial, it boosts the immune system and is useful in the treatment of colds, the flu, herpes, and rheumatoid arthritis.

It is useful in the digestive system, as it is said to absorb toxins and should give you a greater feeling of energy as it helps to balance your blood-sugar level. It has helped in the treatment of people with Chronic Fatigue Syndrome.

- Make an infusion from one to two teaspoons of the dried herb per cup. Olive can have a profound Detox effect, so it is wise to start with a small dose and build up gradually.

Pau D'Arco

The inner bark of pau d'arco is used. It is antibacterial, antiviral, anti-inflammatory, antifungal, anticandida, and so of great help in the treatment of a wide range of parasites. It is found in a number of supplement or herbal combinations aimed at treating candidiasis and fungal infections.

✦✦✦ ✦✦✦

✦ Chapter 9 ✦

Your Liver

YOUR LIVER IS A VITAL ORGAN, performing more chemical tasks than any other organ in your body. It is vital to your health and well-being as well as your ability to deal with and eliminate toxins (see *Liver Detox Plan* for a more detailed discussion). It is a major organ of excretion of toxins and unwanted waste products.

Your liver is the portal of entry for much of your food as it passes from your digestive tract into your bloodstream and disperses throughout your system. While the food that you eat is digested within your digestive system, much of it then finds its way to your liver before being dispersed throughout your body.

Within your digestive system, fats are digested or broken down into smaller molecules. Some fatty acids go directly to your liver. Most of the fats are packaged, at the wall of the small intestine, into manageable packages called chylomicrons that can be transported through your aqueous bloodstream more easily than the fats on their own. As soon as they reach the liver, they are repackaged for even easier transport. They become VLDLs and LDLs, (see p.11), very low and low density lipoproteins respectively. Thus, your liver is responsible for converting fats into forms that can travel throughout the rest of your bloodstream and be delivered to the target organs and cells that need them.

Proteins are broken down within your digestive system into individual amino acids. These are absorbed, carried to your liver, and then rebuilt into the specific proteins that you need. If you have an excess of some amino acids and not enough of others, then to a certain extent, your liver can make the necessary changes.

Carbohydrates are broken down into single sugars in your digestive tract. These are absorbed and transported throughout your body as the simple sugar, glucose. A certain amount of this glucose is always offered to your liver, and if its stores are low, it is taken up and made into glycogen, sometimes called animal starch. In this form, the glucose is stored against such time as your blood sugar level might fall. When this happens, the glycogen is there to feed glucose back into the bloodstream.

The fat-soluble vitamins can be stored in your liver, which in turn facilitates their future transport to the rest of your body. Vitamin A, for instance, is combined with retinol-binding protein, made in the liver, so that it can be carried throughout your bloodstream. Vitamin D is converted from an inactive precursor form to a more active form in your liver.

Small amounts of water-soluble vitamins are stored in your liver. This is why liver, from various animals, is a relatively rich source of these nutrients.

Several minerals, such as copper and iron, are transported throughout your system attached to carrier molecules. These molecules are made in your liver.

Much more than this is done by your liver. It is a significant part of your immune system. Hormones are managed; energy is managed; important blood factors are made; unwanted ammonia is dealt with, as are old hormones; proper cholesterol metabolism is achieved, and hundreds of other actions are accomplished. Above all, from my point of view, the two phases of detoxification, Phase I and Phase II, are accomplished. Phase I of detoxification is the mobilization of toxins. Phase II is the "green-bagging," the packaging of these toxins into a form in which, generally, they can do minimum damage and in which they can most readily be excreted from your body. Thus, it is critically important that your liver is functioning to the very best of its capacity.

Major liver problems include such known diseases as hepatitis, cirrhosis, and jaundice. Liver function tests can tell you if your liver is in serious trouble. However, there are many problems that can occur between perfect health and these serious conditions, problems that will not show up when you do these liver function tests with your doctor. Your liver can be a long way from its optimum best, and yet blood tests may still tell you it is functioning within acceptable, normal levels. This is not good enough if you want to be as healthy as possible and eliminate toxins with maximum efficiency.

Fortunately, the liver is a very forgiving organ, and provided you do right by it and give it all the nutrients and help it needs, plus reduce the amount of unnecessary toxic overload it has to deal with, it can recover from even a pretty bad condition, rebuild itself, and get back into proper action.

Detoxification Via the Digestive Tract

Your liver plays a number of roles in detoxification via your digestive tract. By stimulating normal peristalsis as a result of the effect of the bile that it manufactures and sends out, first to your gallbladder and from there to your small intestine, the liver helps to ensure the proper movement of foods along the digestive tract and thus prevent constipation. This prevents the formation and buildup of toxins in the digestive tract that could then be absorbed into your bloodstream.

This same flow of bile enables you to digest fats properly and prevent an increased load of toxins in your digestive tract.

Systemic Cleansing Effect

Your liver is even more important than this. It is capable of breaking down many of the toxins you consume, inhale, or absorb through your skin. Some of these it can convert into less harmful forms. Some of them it can break down completely. It does this in a great many different ways.

Some of the fat-soluble toxins it converts into water-soluble compounds that can then be excreted either from your liver or via your bladder in urine. Other toxins it actually stores, until such time as it can deal with them. This may put a strain on your liver, but it does reduce the systemic effect they could have if they were allowed to roam freely through your bloodstream. Other toxins are packaged and sent to your storage depots, your adipose tissues where you also store any unwanted fat, as you will know all too well if you think you are overweight.

Other toxins are completely broken down in the liver and reduced to such harmless compounds as carbon dioxide and water.

Clearly your liver is very important. For these reasons, we are paying particular attention to some of the most useful herbs that can benefit it.

Herbs That Can Provide Cleansing Solutions

For a full discussion of what your liver does and how you can help it, consult the *Liver Detox Plan*. Some of the herbs you can use to improve the function of your liver, are medicinal herbs and should be kept and used only when necessary. Others, such as dandelion, can be used on a daily basis to support the liver and keep you healthy.

Many herbs can benefit your liver. Two of the best known are dandelion and milk thistle. They were mentioned briefly in the chapter on your digestive system. It is time now to consider them in greater detail. Dandelion root is readily available as a drink that you can substitute for coffee; the leaves are available as an herbal tea. Milk thistle is available in tincture or tablet form from most health-food stores. Both are frequently included in good combination supplements aimed either at supporting liver function or helping to detox, and when you find them there it is helpful to know what they do. They are discussed below, as are several other herbs that are beneficial to your liver. Some of them you may find in the list of ingredients when you buy a targeted product aimed at improving your liver's function. Others are available, dried or in tincture form, from herbal suppliers.

Dandelion

One of the most readily available herbs that can benefit your liver is the common dandelion. Its Latin name is *Taraxacum officinale* and it belongs to the *Compositae* family. *Taraxos* means "disorder," and *akos* has a Greek root meaning "remedy," so it can be thought of as an herb that has, for a long time, been considered to be capable of bringing about order out of disorder — in this case, order to your liver and kidneys. Nearly all gardens have some plants, and most gardeners wish they didn't. It is generally thought of as a weed and dug up and discarded whenever possible. This is a mistake, for it is an extremely useful and beneficial plant. This gives you a wonderful excuse, if your garden is overrun with this "weed," to say airily to friends: "A weed? Gracious no, this is a valuable herb that I harvest regularly."

If you don't know it, it is easy to recognize. The leaves lie flat, relatively close to the ground, coming from the top of the root and forming a clump from which rises a single hollow stem that contains an acrid white liquid with a bitter flavor. You may have played with this stem as a child, using it as a straw to blow through. On top of this is either the golden yellow flower (or its bud) or the white puffball that says it is about to disperse its seeds and create another hundred or more plants for you. It has a long, tapering root that is often divided and readily breaks off. This means that if you are weeding and simply pull on the plant, you will probably come away with the stem and a handful of leaves and leave some or all of the root behind to come back to haunt you. You need a trowel or hand fork, better still a small version of a full-sized fork. Drive this down beside the plant and gently lift the whole thing, shake off the earth, and take it indoors for cleaning.

If you are interested in a serious Detox, you will keep the leaves. These can be washed and used in salads or, fresh or dried, made into an herbal tea. I have to admit the latter is something of an acquired taste as the leaves are somewhat bitter, but they are excellent for your kidneys. Even better, consider adding some of the fresh leaves to a salad made from a variety of other leaves; you can then lose the flavor among the other bitter greens.

The next step is to clean the root. This is when you will start to wish that it had one large root instead of the bifurcated spindly thing you probably have in your hand. The answer, of course, is to leave it in the ground longer. When friends comment on the vast display of these weeds that you seem to be cultivating, you can tell them you are doing just that. You might even want to keep a part of your garden especially for them, then you can let them grow until they are great granddaddy plants that, when finally dug up, will give you a root large enough to be worth the trouble you are about to take. It must now be cleaned thoroughly and any hard, tough outer skin removed. Chop it as finely as possible — a good, sharp knife is important for this — roast the pieces until they are dried and crisp, and then grind them down to a powder using a small electrical coffee grinder or similar implement. Finally, give them a further roast so the newly exposed surfaces are also toasted. Allow the resultant powder to cool, and store it in an airtight container. When you want your next cup, put three teaspoons of this powder per cup into boiling water, simmer for about fifteen minutes, strain and drink.

If all this sounds like too much trouble, you can hotfoot it down to your nearest health-food store and buy the ground powder there. If you are truly impatient, with no time to spare, you can even buy an instant version. This is the powder, carried on a lactose base. It dissolves instantly on meeting up with a cupful of boiling water and tastes delicious. Unlike regular coffee, it is not bitter, and because of the added lactose, this instant version tastes slightly sweet, and it is possible to enjoy it without the addition of further sugar or honey.

If you are suffering the agonies and difficulties of candidiasis and have been told to avoid lactose, this version is not for you. There is a product that is claimed to be an instant dandelion root tea. It comes in a tea bag with instructions to simply add boiling water. However, nothing I have been able to do — short of boiling the thing for fifteen minutes, and if you are going to do this you might as well buy the ground powder as discussed above — will induce anything to dissolve sufficiently to add either color or flavor to the water.

Do not confuse this instant dandelion coffee with tea bags of dandelion tea. The tea is made from the leaves, and that is a very different matter. As we've said, the leaves are excellent for the kidneys; the root is what want for your liver. The leaves can be picked at any time of year; the roots should be dug up in late summer.

Dandelion contains a variety of active compounds including the carotene form of vitamin A and minerals including potassium. It is a diuretic, hepatic, cholagogue, antirheumatic, laxative, and tonic.

As a diuretic, it aids normal urination and prevents fluid retention, while at the same time and because of its high potassium content, preventing the potassium depletion that occurs with other diuretics. As a hepatic and cholagogue, it helps the liver and stimulates the gallbladder, thus encouraging the flow of bile and the normal digestion of fats; it prevents constipation largely because bile stimulates peristaltic action along the digestive tract. Finally, it helps to reduce the symptoms of rheumatism, and as a general tonic, increases your feeling of well-being.

It offers further benefits to your liver, helping to prevent congestion, inflammation, and jaundice. By stimulating the flow of normal healthy bile that is then transported to your gallbladder, it reduces the risk of gall stones and improves your liver's capacity to Detox and deal with the many toxins to which you are exposed. If you are overweight, its capacity to prevent fluid retention, increase loss of toxins, and tone up your system will make the process of losing weight proceed more smoothly. It works well with milk thistle or bayberry.

Consider replacing your daily cups of tea and/or coffee with cups of Dandelion coffee instead.

DANDELION SALAD

This is a delicious salad if you enjoy bitter leaves. Gather about 1⅓ cups of fresh dandelion leaves and combine with a 1⅓ cups of mixed lettuce leaves, Wash and tear the leaves into smaller sections and place in a salad bowl. Add the leaves of a few springs of lovage and the leaves of a bunch of celery chopped. Make a dressing from olive oil and apple cider vinegar, sweeten with ½ teaspoon honey, and add fresh herbs such as tarragon and origanum. Season to taste with salt and freshly ground black pepper.

Milk Thistle

Milk thistle, or *Silybum marianum,* is another member of the *Compositae* family. It comes originally from the Mediterranean area, so is less likely to be a garden weed in the British Isles than the more common dandelion. Its leaves are glossy green and spiny, and the plant derives its common name from the milk-white veins that run through the leaves and its large purple flowers, bearing some similarities with Scottish thistle.

This time, it is the seeds that are used, rather than the leaves or root, and they can be collected in the late summer or autumn, whenever they are present. Ideally, you should let them dry on the plant, then cover the seed head with a paper bag and knock all the seeds into it.

This is another herb that is readily available, and you will find it in a variety of preparations in health-food stores going under

either name, milk thistle or silymarin. It is a cholagogue, demu-
lent, antioxidant, and galactogogue.

As a cholagogue, it acts on the gallbladder, stimulating the flow
of bile. Silymarin is a selective antioxidant for the liver and so is
particularly valuable for helping to prevent the liver cells from
oxidative damage. Since much of the liver's work as an organ of
detoxification is centered around dealing with free radicals and
other oxidizing substances, this is particularly useful and helps to
protect your liver from harm while it is doing its job. Milk thistle
also acts as a general antioxidant and helps to protect all tissues,
throughout your body from the damage that can be caused by
oxidizing agents.

As a demulcent, it is soothing to the mucous membranes. This
is particularly useful, for our purposes here, when considering
gallstones or inflammation of the gallbladder, as it helps to soothe
and protect the lining of this organ and the lining of the ducts that
lead from it down into the digestive tract, as well as the walls of
the digestive tract itself.

Silybin, another component of milk thistle, is thought to protect
the genetic material within the nuclei of the liver cells and thus
reduce the risk of liver, cancer. It facilitates or improves the
synthesis of proteins in the liver, an important part of both your
liver function in general and of your detox system in particular.
As milk thistle is a galactagogue, meaning it can help stimulate
the flow of breast milk during breast-feeding, it has this extra
benefit for nursing mothers.

Toxins will inevitably stimulate your immune system to attack.
This is turn can generate a variety of anti-inflammatory
compounds, and milk thistle is able to reduce the harmful aspects
of this inflammatory reaction.

In addition to helping you to Detox, milk thistle is useful in the
treatment of all sorts of diseases relating to your liver, including
fatty livers and cirrhosis, especially when the latter is caused by
drinking too much alcohol.

Greater Celandine

Greater celandine is often better known, among therapists, particularly homoepaths, as *Chelidonium*, or *Chelidonium majus*, to give

it its full Latin name. It belongs to the poppy or *Papaveraceae* family and should not be confused with lesser celandine or *Ranunculus ficaria* of the *Ranunculaceae* family. The whole plant is used. If you are growing it, the roots should be dug up in summer or autumn and dried; the leaves and flowers should be picked while the plant is flowering and then dried out of the sun.

It was known to, and used by, the ancient Greeks, chelidon referring to swallows, as the plant flowers in the early summer when these birds arrive and fades when they depart. Pliny talks of using the acrid juice for removing a film from the eyes. The yellow juice from the stem can also be applied to skin cancers, warts, and verrucae and has helped to remove them. Applied to tinea, it can destroy the organism that is causing the problem.

The whole plant contains a number of active ingredients, and it acts as an alterative, antispasmodic, anodyne, cholagogue, diuretic, and purgative.

It is a very useful herb for digestive problems and constipation but should be used cautiously, as large doses can have a dramatic effect. This may sometimes reduce the amount that can be taken, so it is often combined with other liver herbs for a greater effect. This is a medicinal herb and would not normally be taken on a regular basis if there is no apparent need for it, unlike dandelion, which can be eaten or drunk daily.

Chelidonium has been used in the treatment of inflammation of the gallbladder and of gall stones. As an antispasmodic and anodyne, it can help to relax the muscles of the various ducts and reduce cramping pains.

Although not one of the major alteratives or blood cleansers, this attribute is useful, and it would be a good herb to choose if you want to both help your liver and provide a general blood cleansing.

- A normal dosage level of the tincture is ¼ teaspoon three times a day and it is best not to exceed this.

Balmony

Balmony, or *Chelone glabra,* is particularly useful for jaundice and gallbladder problems. It grows in damp places, on the edges of swamps, along rivers, and in wet woodlands. It spreads via the roots and should be contained if you want it to grow without it taking over your garden. The Greek word *chelone* means "tortoise," and the look of the corona is thought to be somewhat like the head of this animal. The dried aerial parts of the plant are used and should be collected and dried during the flowering season, or from July to September. It is an anti-emetic, stimulant, anthelmintic, and gentle laxative.

The main usage for this herb is in conditions of gallbladder problems, where there is inflammation of the gallbladder, either due to infection or to the presence of gravel or stones, and in the treatment of jaundice. It is used in the treatment of stones, particularly when these stones are sufficiently large that they block the flow of bile. When this happens, the bile backs up into the liver and is dispersed throughout the bloodstream, causing the typical yellowing of the skin seen in jaundice. It combines well with golden seal for this condition.

It is also an excellent herb for the liver in general and for the whole digestive system. It stimulates appetite and the flow of digestive juices. In this way, it improves most aspects of digestion and, because of its action on the liver and gallbladder and on the flow of bile, it gently stimulates normal peristalsis and relieves constipation. In the treatment of constipation, it works particularly well when combined with golden seal. It has been used in the treatment of dyspepsia or heartburn, nausea and colic.

As an anthelmintic, it would be a good herb to choose if there is any possibility of worms being present.

Externally it has been used in the treatment of inflamed breasts, painful ulcers, and hemorrhoids. It can be applied as a poultice or as a cream.

- An infusion can be made by steeping two teaspoons of the dried herb per cup in boiled water for 10 to 15 minutes. If you are using the tincture, the usual dose is ¼ teaspoon taken three times a day.

Barberry

Barberry, also known as *Berberis vulgaris*, is a common garden shrub that grows slowly. The remedy is made from the bark of the root and stem plus the berries. It is antiseptic, cholagogue, anti-emetic, bitter, tonic, and laxative.

This is an excellent herb for the whole digestive system and the liver. We covered it briefly in the section on the stomach, as it helps to get that organ off to a good start. It demands attention here, as it is very beneficial to the liver and gallbladder. It can be used for digestive problems that also include such gallbladder problems as nausea and biliousness, an inflamed gallbladder and gallstones, or for liver problems — both mild, and those severe enough to cause jaundice. Because it stimulates the flow of bile, it is able to give a gentle boost to the peristaltic action of the lower digestive system and act as a mild laxative.

Barberry is quite effective against a number of microorganisms including those that cause malaria and the fungus *Candida albicans*. It is suggested that you do not use this herb if you are pregnant.

- When making a decoction, allow one teaspoonful of the dried root per cup, and pour on boiling water. Alternatively, take ¼ to ½ teaspoon of the tincture two or three times a day. If you are using the berries, extract the juice.

Black Root

Black root, or *Leptandra virginica,* from the *Scrophulariaceae* family was used by the Seneca Indians. As a result of their knowledge, it was in time introduced into European herbal medicine. The root is used, but time is required, as it should be dug up in the autumn and then stored for a year before being used as a remedy.

It acts as a cholagogue, mild cathartic, diaphoretic, and anti-spasmodic. This is a specific herb for the liver and gallbladder and any problems that can stem from their malfunction. It is used in the treatment of cholecystitis or inflamed gallbladder and for liver congestion that can lead to jaundice. Since these problems can reduce the flow of bile into the digestive tract, black root can also be used for constipation. It works well with barberry and dandelion for the treatment of liver congestion.

While the dried root is a mild cathartic, the fresh root can be a violent one and is also sometimes an emetic. It should be used with care.

- Allow one teaspoon of the ground dried root per cup, and simmer for 10 minutes. If you prefer the tincture, then ¼ to ½ teaspoon taken three times a day is the usual dose.

Blue Flag

Blue flag, or *Iris versicolor,* from the *Iridaceae* family is not only a beautiful flower, but the rhizome is an excellent remedy. It grows in wet and swampy ground and is collected in autumn when the flower has died down. It has a range of uses and acts as an anti-inflammatory, alterative, cholagogue, diuretic and laxative.

This means that it is an excellent herb to use in a Detox Regime. Not only does it improve elimination via your colon and kidneys, it improves liver function, is a good blood cleanser and can be used to improve your skin. It has been found to be helpful in the treatment of eczema and psoriasis but particularly in the treatment of acne and similar skin eruptions. For this latter purpose it combines well with burdock and yellow dock.

- To make an infusion allow ½ to 1 teaspoon of the dried herb to a cup of boiling water. If you are using the tincture the recommended dose is ¼ to ½ teaspoon taken three times a day.

Boldo

Boldo, also known as *Peumus boldo,* is another herb that refutes the rumor that herbs are small and delicate plants. It is a small shrub-like tree that is indigenous to South America, particularly Chile. The leaves are used and, since they are evergreen, can be gathered at any time and then dried. The herb is a cholagogue, diuretic, hepatic, and sedative. Other parts of the plant are useful, too; the fruit is eaten, and the bark used for tanning.

It is particularly useful for gallbladder inflammation and gallstones, and works well with fringetree bark for this purpose. However, it is also useful in the treatment of cystitis, as it is mildly antiseptic and demulcent, and in fluid retention. This means that if you are in need of a liver herb and also suffer from cystitis, this would be a particularly good one to choose.

- You can make an infusion, in which case allow 1 teaspoon of the dried leaves to one cup of boiling water, or take ¼ teaspoon of the tincture three times a day.

Fringetree Bark

Fringetree, an evocative name, was mentioned above. It is also known as *Chionanthus virginicus*, which is somewhat more difficult to pronounce, and belongs to the *Oleaceae* family. Again we are dealing with a tree, not a small plant, and this time it is the root bark that is used. The root should be dug up in spring or autumn, the bark cleaned and then peeled. It acts as a cholagogue, hepatic, alterative, diuretic, tonic, and laxative.

Its main action is on the liver and gallbladder, where it is used to treat gallstones, gallbladder inflammation, and liver problems with jaundice. It will also, of course, help to normalize bowel movements. It works well in combination with some of the other liver herbs we have discussed here, including boldo, barberry, wahoo, and wild yam.

As it is also an alterative, it offers this additional benefit in a Detox Regime.

- If you are making an infusion, use one to two teaspoons of the dried herb per cup of boiling water. If you prefer the tincture, take ¼ teaspoon three times a day.

Golden Seal

Golden seal, which was discussed in detail earlier (see p.93) is not generally thought of as a specific for the liver. Many other herbs would be chosen first if you have a specific liver or gallbladder problem. However, it has many uses and offers many benefits to the digestive system and mucous membranes, is active against many parasites, helps to prevent constipation, and combines well with so many herbs that it should be considered in any Detox Regime where you are trying to stimulate liver function, both in relation to the digestive tract and in regard to the liver's role in systemic detoxification.

Due to its beneficial effect on mucous membranes, it is a beneficial part of any treatment for gallstones or gravel, where there will also be damage to the membranes lining the ducts.

Consider adding it to some of the liver herbs discussed in this section.

Vervain

Vervain, or *Verbena officinalis*, from the *Labiatae* family, also has the delightful common name of Herb of Grace. It has small lilac flowers that can be found growing wild at roadsides and in hedgerows. There is a possible Celtic derivation to its name; ferfaenm from "fer" to "drive away," and "faen" or "stone."

It should be collected just before the flowers open, usually in July, and should then be dried rapidly. It acts as an astringent, nervine, tonic, sedative, antispasmodic, diaphoretic, possible galactogue, and hepatic.

It has several uses in the process of detoxification. It can be used as a mouthwash to help protect against caries and gum disease. This is often important during a Detox Regime, as many people will report a furry tongue and bad taste in their mouth as they start the process of both reducing the intake of toxins and encouraging the activation and removal of stored toxins. It may also be that mouth, gum, or throat infections are present and constitute part of your motivation for going on a Detox Regime in the first place.

As a diaphoretic, it will help to increase perspiration and the loss of toxins in this way. Detox does not necessarily lead to a raised temperature, but, on the other hand, an increase in temperature is one of the body's defenses against invading organisms and infections. When it occurs, it is good to encourage the loss of toxins in this way.

As a hepatic, of course, it has a direct action on the liver and gallbladder, stimulates their normal function, and can be useful in the treatment of jaundice. However, it is not a major hepatic herb and should be used in combination with some of the others discussed here.

If you are not only toxic but depressed as well, a not uncommon occurrence, then vervain is useful here, too. It is used in the treatment of depression, particularly after debilitating illnesses or an infectious disease. In these situations, it acts well in combination with skullcap, oats, and lady's slipper.

- To make an infusion, use between 1 and 3 teaspoons of dried herb per cup; if taking the tincture, the normal dose is ½ to 1 teaspoon three times day.

Wahoo

Wahoo — even its name sounds interesting, as does its Latin name, *Euonymus atropurpureus*. We again move away from the idea of a delicate green herb. It is the bark of the root that is used, and this should be dug up in autumn, although the bark of the stem can be used as an alternative.

The herb acts as a hepatic stimulant, cholagogue, laxative, diuretic, tonic, and alterative. We discussed it briefly when dealing with problems of the colon and with constipation; however, its main role is due to its action on the liver. It is one of the most useful liver herbs, along with dandelion and milk thistle, and is helpful in the treatment of all liver and gallbladder problems including jaundice, gallstones, and gallbladder inflammation or pain. However, it is also useful if none of these problems are present but you just feel sluggish and "liverish," as it is a general tonic and toner for the liver and encourages it back into action.

It is also, of course, useful in the treatment of associated problems such as indigestion and constipation and as an alterative it is useful in the treatment of skin problems associated with poor liver function.

- You can make a decoction by using between half and a whole teaspoonful of the dried herb per cup. If you are taking the tincture, the generally recommended dose is between ten drops and one teaspoon three times a day.

Yellow Dock

It is the root of yellow dock or *Rumex crispus* from the *Polyconaceae* family that is used as a remedy, and this should be dug up in late summer or early autumn. It an alterative, cholagogue, laxative, and antiviral.

Do not be put off by its place at the end of the alphabet and so at the end of this chapter. This is an extremely useful herb.

It is generally thought of as a blood-cleansing herb useful for skin problems and helping in the treatment of acne and psoriasis. Thus, it is a valuable herb in any Detox Regime. However, it has other uses in a Detox Regime, as it is a mild liver stimulant and has been used in the treatment of jaundice. It also acts on the colon, producing a mild laxative effect.

If you are trying to improve your skin and deal with signs of toxicity there, then it works well in combination with burdock and poke root. If you are also constipated and want to support your liver, then use it in conjunction with dandelion root.

- Make a decoction by using one to two teaspoons of the dried herb per cup. For the tincture, ¼ to ½ teaspoon can be taken three times a day.

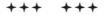

✦ CHAPTER 10 ✦

Your Immune System

WE HAVE, SO FAR, DISCUSSED THE HERBS you can use to help your digestive tract and your liver. A healthy lifestyle and digestive system will help to ensure that you do not take in unwanted toxins. A healthy lining to your digestive system, and avoiding problems that could result from a leaky gut if the lining of your digestive tract is damaged, is another important defense against the intake of toxins, as is the prevention of constipation and the formation of new toxins within your digestive system.

Now it is time to move on to your next line of defense, your immune system. If toxins have been absorbed and you have unwanted and harmful organisms in your system, then it is up to your immune system to tackle them.

Your immune system is your defense against the world. It is your immune system that recognizes what is you and what is not you. It protects what is you and fights what is not. However, its role is even more subtle than this. Think about it. Substances you take in as food are "not you," yet your immune system must allow you to take them in and use them. It should not treat food as a foreign invader. Normally it manages this process very well. Sometimes it makes mistakes, and this is when you become allergic to certain foods.

How does your immune system deal with toxins and pathogens? It has a variety of ways of doing this. There are specific cells, your white cells, that are part of the immune system. Most of them are free to migrate and roam throughout not only your bloodstream but your tissues as well. Put simply, they recognize something, such as a bacteria, as foreign, they engulf it, and then they destroy it.

There are also proteins known as antibodies. Each time a foreign substance, by definition called an antigen, enters your body, an opposing antibody is made whose job it is to deal with and destroy or deactivate the antigen.

When a foreign substance or organism enters your body, your immune system gets to work. An inflammation of some sort may develop while this is happening — the typical symptoms of which are redness, heat, swelling, and pain. If your immune system fails to act properly, you will succumb to the infection or feel the adverse effect of the toxins.

Many things can harm your immune system. It can be overworked, as can happen when you are exposed to a wide variety and a large amount of toxins. It will suffer if you do not provide all the nutrients it needs. If you are emotionally stressed and challenged, it gets called into play and can then become exhausted.

We know, for instance, that when you are sad, you are more inclined to succumb to an infection such as the flu than when you are happy. It is not uncommon to find that if one partner of an elderly couple dies, the other one becomes ill soon after, commonly with pneumonia, and may also die. We now know that the stress of the first death leads, in the survivor, to a marked drop in the number of white blood cells, the defense cells of their immune system. This then leaves them vulnerable to any infection that is around.

The medical philosophy is inclined to embrace the idea that you get ill because a bug invades you. If the bug can be killed, then you will get well again, hence the use of antibiotics, often as the only therapy that is offered.

The naturopathic philosophy is quite different, essentially the opposite in fact. It says that when you are in good health, you can ward off all, or at least most, bugs and deal with a wide range of toxins. It is only when your defenses are weakened that the bugs, the bacteria, and so forth can even get in and make any impact. Thus, the naturopathic approach, and the approach adopted here, is to build up your immune system to help you keep the toxins, the microorganisms, and other infectious agents out. Nonetheless, and in addition to this, there are many herbs that are antimicrobial and can help to decimate the invading organisms, while at the same time helping to rebuild your immune system. We will start off by looking at some of these.

Antimicrobials

Antimicrobials are, as the name implies, substances or herbs that act against invading microorganisms. To this extent, they can be considered to be somewhat like antibiotics. However, you will discover, as you read through this section, that that is not all they do. In general, they also act in a number of beneficial and positive ways both on your immune system and on various other parts and systems of your body.

Cat's Claw

Cat's claw has nothing to do with cats. It is a plant that goes by the Latin name of *Uncaria tomentosa*, and is a vine found growing around rain forest trees in the Amazon valley of South America. The inner red bark of this vine is used in herbal medicine and contains at least four alkaloids that stimulate the immune system and the engulfing of toxins by some of your white blood cells.

Cat's claw supports the action of the immune system in several ways. It is an anti-inflammatory, antioxidant, antiviral, antitumor, antimutagenic, immune-stimulant. In simpler terms, this means that it helps your body to resist the effect of viruses and also of oxidizing agents and free radicals that could cause cells to mutate or develop into cancerous cells. It reduces the tendency to inflammation, while also encouraging your white blood cells to engulf and destroy harmful organisms and toxins.

For our purpose, this means in particular that it is a useful boost to improving your overall health and that it accomplishes this by helping you to avoid infections and inflammations.

In the digestive system, it helps to rebalance the intestinal flora in favor of the beneficial microorganisms, encouraging them and inhibiting the growth of harmful ones. It has been considered to be a general digestive cleanser and has been used in the treatment of gastritis, ulcers, candidiasis, parasites and other intestinal flora imbalances, diverticulitis, hemorrhoids, leaky gut, and Crohn's disease.

It is often recommended as a general cleansing herb for a wide range of toxic poisonings, and can help to reduce allergic reactions.

It can also help to reduce skin infections and is useful as a wash for cuts and abrasions; it's used in the treatment of allergies, including those, such as eczema, that can affect the skin, and it is beneficial in your body's defense against herpes or cold sores and in the prevention of skin cancers.

Other than Detox, it has further benefits. It is helpful in the prevention or treatment of asthma, arthritis, cardiovascular problems such as "sticky blood" (platelet aggregation), high blood pressure, poor circulation, and thrombosis. It helps to inhibit plaque formation and has been recommended for both the prevention and treatment of heart attacks, strokes, and angina.

Furthermore, it can help to reduce the experience of stress by helping to relax the tension of voluntary muscles.

- This herb can be used as a preventive if you think an infection is likely; or simply for a short period to give your immune system a boost. For these purposes, the usual dose is ¼ to ½ teaspoon of the dried herb a day. If you are using it to treat a particular problem, then this can be increased to ½ to 1 tablespoon a day. If you want to take more than this, it would be wise to get professional advice. It is also suggested that you should get advice before using this herb if you are pregnant, breast-feeding, or have had a transplant.

Echinacea

Echinacea angustifolia, one of the *Compositae,* is native to North America and used by the American Indians for wounds, bites and stings, sore gums, colds and other infections, and arthritis. Echinacea is also one of the most important herbs for the support of your immune system and is commonly available in most health-food stores.

The roots should be lifted in the autumn. They act as an antibacterial, antifungal, antiviral, and alterative.

Put simply, this means that it is a blood cleanser, and it fights invading organisms. It is an extremely important and effective anti-microbial acting against many different types of bacteria, viruses, and molds and can be used in the treatment of many related health problems throughout the body. Thus, it plays a particularly important role in any Detox Regime that has to be effective against microorganisms and viruses.

It acts with and helps your immune system in so many different ways that they are worth listing:

- It stimulates cellular immunity by stimulating the activity of T-lymphocytes, a sub-group of your defensive white cells.
- It stimulates the production of macrophages. These are large cells that consume pathogenic or harmful microorganisms and toxins.
- It stimulates the production of complement, a substance found in the blood that causes the destruction of toxic bacteria.
- It protects the body by stimulating the cellular production of interferon, a substance that helps to prevent viruses from entering your cells and thus prevents the outbreak of viral infections.
- It activates the reticulo-endothelium layer system. This is a network of cells found throughout your body that plays important roles within your immune system and that helps to reduce inflammation.
- It increases the production of antibodies, particularly the alpha, beta, and gamma globulins. These antibodies are proteins produced by your own cells in response to the invasion of toxic substances, known collectively as antigens. Individual antibodies are programd to fight specific antigens.
- It stimulates phagocytosis, the process by which toxins are engulfed by cells of your defense system, preliminary to the substances either being destroyed or excreted.
- It stimulates the production of granulomatous tissue, which is produced in response to the presence of toxic microorganisms.
- Finally, it stimulates the activity of the lymphatic system, thus encouraging the removal of waste material, particularly from infected areas.

With all these beneficial activities, it is hardly surprising to find it being recommended for a wide range of conditions. It is used as a mouthwash for pyrrhoea and gingivitis, and externally as a cleansing wash for cuts and wounds. In candidiasis, it is used, in conjunction with specific antifungals, to rebuild the immune system.

The ground substance of your connective tissues, the fine tissues that hold the various parts of your body together, contains a substance called hyaluronic acid and its derivatives. These connective tissues can be broken down by the action of hyaluronidase, an enzyme that can be produced by pathogenic or harmful organisms. This enzyme is inhibited by echinacea, which in this way can prevent damage and encourage healing. Thus, it is useful in the treatment and detoxing of any situations that involve connective tissue damage.

Typically, echinacea is thought of when there are coughs and colds, influenza, catarrhal situations such as bronchitis, laryngitis or tonsillitis, boils, septicaemia, and other infections, including cystitis, which we will be considering in the next section.

The decoction can be made by allowing one to two teaspoons of the root per cup and simmering the mixture for 15 minutes. This can be drunk three times a day. If you are using the tincture, you can take from ¼ to ½ teaspoon three times a day. The non-alcoholic forms of this herb are preferred for actions affecting the immune system.

Eucalyptus

Eucalyptus is discussed in detail in the chapter on the skin (p.191), but it also deserves a mention here.

It supports the immune system and is a even a mild antimalarial, though not as good as cinchona. It is excellent for a variety of respiratory problems such as mucus, catarrh, nasal congestion, sore throat, coughs, colds, or flu. Use it as a chest- or throat-rub or as a mouthwash and gargle.

It is helpful for asthma if inhaled. Add a few drops to boiling water for this purpose, and inhale the steam.

Garlic

Garlic, or *Allium sativum*, a member of the *Liliaceae* family, has so many uses it is difficult to know where to start. The bulb should be harvested in the autumn, as you would if growing it as a vegetable, when the leaves are beginning to wither. It has multiple actions and is an anthelmintic, antifungal, antimicrobial, antiseptic, antiviral, antiparasitic, detoxicant, diaphoretic, cholagogue, and lipid-lowering hypotensive. Clearly it has a vast amount to offer us in the development of a Detox Regime. Let's look at its various roles in more detail.

The first six roles all involve its activity on a range of microorganisms or pathogens, so clearly it is of great benefit to your immune system. As it can also destroy pathogens in the gut, it may even decrease the work your immune system has to do. It is thought that its destructive effect on harmful organisms comes about because it can block the synthesis of the genetic material, the DNA and RNA of the organisms concerned. Any herb that can block the replication of DNA within a cell can have a serious effect on that cell. It can block the actions of the cell or organism and it can stop the cell, and hence the microorganism or pathogen, dividing and so multiplying. Once this is accomplished, then the potential infection is successfully curtailed. There is evidence for specific results of this activity.

As an antibacterial, garlic has been shown to inhibit such pathogens as *Giardia lamblia, Streptococcus sp.,* and *Salmonella sp.* These may be unfamiliar names and creatures to you, but it is sometimes worth having a more detailed understanding of just what an herb can do, and it can give you more confidence than the simple statement that "garlic can destroy harmful organisms." These particular organisms can cause quite a range of harmful effects.

As an antifungal, garlic is active against *Candida albicans*, so anyone suffering from this unpleasant and often persistent problem should make good use of garlic, both raw in salads and salad dressings, and in cooking, as well as taking it in supplement form. This will help in the treatment of fungal infections on the skin, such as athlete's foot, fungal infections under fingernails, and in other warm and damp places where its growth is encouraged. It's also useful in the treatment of vaginitis and vaginal thrush. For skin problems such as athlete's foot, garlic powder can be applied directly to the area. Because you are working on a mold that likes damp places, the powder is more effective than any type of solution. You may be accused of not washing your socks, but at least you will solve the problem.

As an antiviral, it is helpful in the treatment of Herpes hominis type I, and flu.

Clearly, garlic will give your whole immune system a boost and help it to fight off a range of infections, both externally and internally. Increase your intake of garlic during such infectious conditions as flu, colds, sinusitis, whooping cough, bronchitis, and bronchial asthma. In all such infections, it combines well with echinacea.

Garlic will help to get rid of parasites in the gut, not only of *Candida albicans* but, working as an anthelmintic, of worms and other parasites.

It has additional benefits, not necessarily part of a Detox Regime, but useful nonetheless. Because of its lipid-lowering action, it is helpful in maintaining the health of the cardiovascular system, keeping down cholesterol and triglyceride levels. It also helps to maintain normal blood sugar levels and so has all these benefits to offer to someone with diabetes.

The best way to take garlic is to use it as a food. Eat one or two cloves a day, more if desired, or take it as oil-filled capsules. Keep in mind that the compounds that give garlic its characteristic taste and odor also provide many of its health benefits, so "deodorized" garlic products almost certainly are less effective than the nondeodorized forms. You can always chew parsley or mint afterwards if the smell becomes a problem.

Some of the beneficial compounds in garlic begin to break down when it is crushed, so eat it as fresh as possible. If you want a concentrated form, use one that has been processed by removing water and some of the fiber but still provides garlic in its intact form.

GARLIC WITH SPINACH

I use the relationship of the terms advisedly, for this is one way of consuming prodigious amounts of garlic and thoroughly enjoying the experience.

Allow three cups of spinach leaves per person, wash the leaves and shake dry, put into an empty saucepan, and place over a low heat, allowing the leaves to cook in their own steam. When thoroughly cooked, drain the leaves and squeeze out any excess fluid. While that was cooking, you should have been heating either butter or olive oil over a low heat.

Allow at least three or four *huge* cloves of garlic per person, more, many more, if they are only small cloves, and more still if you enjoy the flavor and are either alone or sharing the meal with the people or person with whom you will be spending the next few hours. Crush this garlic and allow it to soften gently in the butter or oil. Do not overheat this; you do not want to "fry" the garlic.

When all is cooked, add the garlic mixture to the spinach (not the other way around, as you do not want to "fry" the spinach), and serve. It goes well with scrambled eggs or an omelette or with any meat or poultry dish.

You would be well advised to serve this with a parsley salad and finish the meal with peppermint tea to try to at least control some of the odors that will emanate. Never mind, your immune system will thank you.

Licorice

The basic information on licorice was given in the section on the colon (p.110) and for dealing with constipation. However, it was originally better known as an herb for the immune system.

It is a a demulcent, emollient, pectoral, and is particularly useful in the treatment and prevention of infections of the lungs. It achieves its results in several ways. It improves the action of the cells that are responsible for engulfing and destroying toxins and invading organisms. It increases your white blood cell production of interferon, thus helping to protect you from viral infections, and it has a broad spectrum antimicrobial effect.

Use it if you suffer from catarrh, excess or very viscous mucus, coughs and colds, bronchitis, or other chest infections. You will commonly find it in a number of cough remedies, be they herbal tinctures, lozenges, or throat pastilles, where it is selected for its soothing effect as well as for its flavor which often hides the less appealing flavor of some of the other ingredients. Gargle with it for sore throats or laryngitis.

In all these ways, licorice can be helpful if you need to clear up lung infections and eliminate toxins from the lungs. It works well for this purpose with herbs such as coltsfoot, pleurisy root, and horehound.

Myrrh

Myrrh, best known for its role as one of the gifts of the three wise men, is *Commiphora molmol* of the *Burseraceae* family. It is a bush that grows in dry parts of Arabia and East Africa.

The gum or resin is used and contains essential oils. It is anticatarrhal, antimicrobial, astringent, expectorant, and vulnerary so clearly has a great deal to offer to your immune system. It is particularly effective in clearing up problems of the digestive tract. Use it as a mouthwash for pyorrhoea, gingivitis, and mouth ulcers. Myrrh is a component of many toothpastes found in health-food stores and is useful in the treatment of gum problems.

Make a gargle from the tincture for such conditions as sinusitis, pharyngitis, laryngitis, colds and the flu, and remember to swallow it afterwards rather than spitting it out, as this will add to its beneficial action. For skin conditions such as boils, cuts, and other wounds, apply it locally for its antimicrobial action, and take it internally for the systemic benefit this will give to your immune actions.

It has also been beneficial for such systemic infections as glandular fever. It combines well with echinacea for colds and other infections. If you are applying it externally, it works well with witch hazel. It is an ingredient in several toothpastes sold in health food stores.

- It is difficult to make infusions or decoctions with this herb, as the resin does not dissolve easily. It does, however, dissolve in alcohol, so the tincture is effective. Between ¼ to ½ teaspoon can be taken three times a day.

Nasturtium

Anyone with the tiniest garden can grow nasturtiums. Sow a few seeds, and within a few weeks you will have a wonderful display that will come up year after year.

In Latin it is *Tropaeolum majus*, one of the *Tropaeolaceae*. The flowers, seeds, and leaves are used and contain vitamin C. Nasturtium is a powerful antimicrobial, particularly an antibacterial, and can be used to give the general immune system a boost.

Use it to clear up colds, the flu, and bronchitis. It may be of help for infections such as cystitis and pelvic inflammatory disease, and it can be applied directly to any broken skin to prevent or treat infections.

The best results are obtained when the fresh plant is used, and this is easy to do. The flowers, leaves, and seeds can all be used in cooking or added to salads. The leaves and flowers can be made into a poultice to clear up external skin problems. The dried seed cases can be pickled and used instead of capers.

- If you want to use the tincture, then take ¼ to ½ teaspoon three times a day.

NASTURTIUM SALAD WITH DRESSING

Toss together a combination of salad leaves, a handful of nasturtium leaves, and nasturtium flowers. For the dressing, combine olive oil and fresh lemon juice, add finely chopped nasturtium leaves, and a small sprig of sweet cicely, chopped. Season to taste, pour over the salad, and toss.

Schizandra

The berry of *Schizandra chinensis* is used. It is antioxidant, antihepatotoxic; a central nervous system, respiratory, immune system and uterine tonic; and improves lipid and carbohydrate metabolism.

This needs some explaining. Schizandra is an antioxidant. Why is that important? You need oxygen, your body needs oxygen, yet at the same time oxygen is one of the most dangerous substances around you. To resolve this seeming paradox, it is important to understand what happens to the food you eat and how energy is generated.

All foods, be they fats, proteins, or carbohydrates, contain carbon, hydrogen, and a (relatively) small amount of oxygen, in the form of triglycerides, fatty acids, and glycerol, amino acids and glucose. You want the energy these substances contain.

Your first step is to digest the foods and absorb the glucose, fatty acids, and amino acids that are released. The second step is to release the energy bound within these smaller molecules and make this available for every cell in your body. This is done by "burning" these fuels, just like you burn wood or coal to release the heat energy locked within them. In both cases, this "burning" needs oxygen, the reactions are oxidations, and in both cases the end or waste products are carbon dioxide and water.

Thus, you need oxygen to "burn" the foods you eat. Yet what is your body, your flesh and blood, but a mixture of the same components, of fats, proteins, and carbohydrates, which could also be burnt or oxidized and broken down by these same reactions. It is vitally important that you are able to oxidize the foods you eat, but equally important that you do not oxidize your own body. If you do, the end result is many of the diseases of the human body, particularly the degenerative diseases, and more particularly, cancer.

This is why antioxidants are so important. They protect you from the potentially harmful effect of oxygen, while allowing that same oxygen to be the agent that releases the food's energy so vital to your cells. You will notice that in the process, it improves the metabolism of fats and carbohydrates. These effects are inter-linked.

As an antihepatotoxic, schizandra helps to protect your liver from the damaging effect of toxins so that, in turn, it can do its work of protecting the rest of your body.

For our purposes here, it is an invaluable and deep immune stimulant, having a more fundamental and general effect on the whole immune system than the other herbs described in this section. This effect incorporates its antioxidant and antihepato-toxic roles, and as such, it deserves a place in any Detox Regime.

There is more. Schizandra is a tonic to your central nervous system, giving you an energy boost and helping to clear out a fuzzy head, a tonic to your respiratory system, and a uterine tonic.

- To make a decoction of the berries, allow one to three teaspoons per cup.

Thyme

Thyme was discussed earlier, in the chapter on the digestive tract (p.89). However, it is worth remembering that it is, among other things, an antifungal and antimicrobial, and can give significant support to your immune system. Since it is also a culinary herb, it is easy to add to your regular intake.

Others

There are many, many other herbs that will help your immune system. They include all that are alterative, antimicrobial, antifungal, antiviral, anthelmintics, and vermifuges. The ones I have included here, such as cat's claw, echinacea, and garlic, are particularly powerful. Garlic, nasturtium, and thyme have the added benefit of being readily available and easy to incorporate into your diet, and schizandra will give your overall immune system a boost at the deepest level.

Diaphoretics and Febrifuges

When your immune system is in action or you have an infection, it is common to find that your temperature rises. This is beneficial and helpful, not something to be overcome. With each degree rise of temperature, the enzymes that catalyze the reactions your immune system is performing act many times more rapidly. This means that your increased temperature is not so much a final result of the infection as a feature caused by your immune system to make its job easier.

As a result, this means that you should not immediately try to stop or suppress the fever and lower your temperature. You should certainly not try to do this with drugs that can block the process. Instead, welcome the temperature as a sign of the activity and effectiveness of your immune system, then provide the right herbs and support necessary to stimulate immune activity and bring about a proper resolution as rapidly and gently as possible.

The group of herbs to use here are the diaphoretics or febrifuges, and to some extent their roles overlap. The diaphoretics increase perspiration to aid elimination of toxins through the skin.

Febrifuges help to lower your body's temperature, but in a constructive way. Instead of suppressing the fever, febrifuges encourage the process and increase its efficiency. As a result, they reduce the amount of time needed for the infection to be beaten, and hasten the moment when your temperature can return to normal of its own accord — its job being done and the toxins killed, eliminated, or both.

Some of the more common or more useful diaphoretics and febrifuges are discussed below:

Angelica

Angelica has a long history both as an herb and as a food. *Angelica archangelica*, an *Umbelliferae*, is generally thought of as a food today, the green-sugared confection being used to decorate cakes and desserts; it is also a flavoring for some liqueurs. In fact, it is the stems' leaves and seeds that are used in confectionery, and the root and leaves that are used in herbal medicine.

The leaves are collected in summer, and the roots dug up in early autumn. They contain essential oils, and the herb is carminative, stomachic, antispasmodic, expectorant, diuretic, and diaphoretic.

As a diaphoretic, it is useful in the treatment of coughs, bronchitis, pleurisy, colds, flu, and fevers in general, increasing the loss of toxins. At the same time as taking it internally for lung infections, possibly in conjunction with coltsfoot and horehound, it can be used as a compress on the chest.

It offers additional benefits, relieving flatulence and colic, being a useful antiseptic in the treatment of cystitis, and reducing the pain and inflammation of rheumatism.

• Make a decoction allowing one teaspoonful of the root per cup, simmer this for a few minutes, and then leave to infuse. Alternatively, take ½ to 1 teaspoon of the tincture three times a day. If you must eat something sweet, even the candied stems do have some benefit.

Boneset

Boneset should not be confused with comfrey, which is sometimes given the same name and is indeed helpful in the treatment of broken bones. This plant, also known as thoroughwort, or *Eupatorium perfoliatum*, is a *Compositae*. It is a perennial herb that grows in low-lying meadows and damp ground and was known by the American Indians as "ague-weed."

The leaves and flowers should be collected in summer as soon as the plant flowers. The herb is diaphoretic, aperient, tonic, and antispasmodic.

It is one of the best herbs for dealing with flu and the common cold, helping to increase perspiration and reduce the severity of the fever and to help relieve the general body aches and pains, in much the same way it is also beneficial in conditions of rheumatism where there is spastic muscle involvement.

It is also helpful in a Detox Regime by acting gently but beneficially in cases of constipation.

- Make a decoction from one to two teaspoons per cup and drink this, as hot as you can, every half hour or so until the fever abates. Use it in combination with cayenne and ginger if you are impatient, or with elder and yarrow for a more gentle result. If you use the tincture, take between ½ and 1 teaspoon three times a day.

Catnip

Catnip is an easy herb to grow, can be found in many gardens, and as its name might imply, is loved by cats who can often be found sitting on it or even eating it. The leaves and flowers of *Nepeta cataria*, a *Labiatae*, should be collected in summer. It is an astringent, carminative, strong diaphoretic, antispasmodic, and sedative.

Its main use is in the treatment of colds, flu, and bronchitis, but is also helpful in the treatment of flatulence, dyspepsia, colic, and nervous tension.

- An infusion is made from one to two teaspoons of the dried leaves per cup. The tincture dose is ½ to 1 teaspoon taken three times a day.

Cayenne

Cayenne has already been discussed earlier. However, it is also a diaphoretic, as anyone will know who has eaten a very hot curry. "Feed a cold and starve a fever" is an old saying, so if you feel like a curry next time you have a cold, your body could be telling you just what it needs.

Elder

Elder, or *Sambucus nigra* (*Caprifoliaceae*), has already been mentioned briefly as a laxative (p.109). However, it is probably better known by its other common name of sambucus, as a help when you have a cold or flu.

Those living in the country will be familiar with this tree, as it intertwines with everything else growing nearby. The berries are diaphoretic and a rich source of vitamin C and a variety of associated bioflavonoids; the leaves and flowers are also diaphoretic. In addition, sambucol, which is extracted from the berries, is antiviral. It achieves this by binding with viruses before they enter your cells and thus prevents their entry. If a virus cannot enter a cell, then it cannot use the cell's reproductive machinery to make copies of itself, so the virus cannot multiply. In this way, it is prevented from doing harm. Sambucol also stimulates the reproduction of lymphocytes, some of your important immune system white cells, and is an antioxidant.

Such is the power of sambucol that it can be used in the treatment not only of colds and the flu, but of the herpes virus and the Epstein-Barr virus, and has been suggested as part of the naturopathic approach to the treatment of AIDS.

- Make an infusion allowing two teaspoons of the blossoms and leaves per cup, and drink this three times a day. If you prefer the juice, boil the berries in water, crush, add honey, dilute to taste, and drink a cupful three times a day. The tincture dose is ¼ to ½ teaspoon three times a day. The berries can also be made into jams, jellies, soft drinks, and wine.

ELDERBERRY DESSERT

By making this dessert, you can indulge a (slightly) sweet tooth in the knowledge that you are adding to your intake of vitamin C, and if you have the flu or some other infection, that you are helping your defenses to deal with the virus.

Gather seven cups of fresh elderberries, crush, and then sieve to extract the juice. Peel and core an apple, and put it and the elder juice in a blender. Add two cups of natural yogurt and the juice of one lemon, sweeten with honey, and blend. You will want to adjust the proportions until you get a result that pleases you. Elderberries are rich in flavor and you may prefer more yogurt or lemon juice.

This can be served on its own as a dessert or with other fresh fruits as a dressing. Omit the yogurt and use it as a sauce to serve with turkey or some other meat dish.

Ginger

Ginger was discussed in the chapter on the digestive tract (p.88). It is also worth a brief mention here, as it is a diaphoretic and helpful when you have a temperature and want to increase natural and healing perspiration. Try adding boiling water to a few slices of fresh ginger, sweeten with honey if you wish, and sip this throughout the day. It will help to relieve your symptoms and speed your recovery.

Hyssop

The leaves and flowers of *Hyssopus officinalis*, a *Labiatae*, are collected in late summer. They are antispasmodic, carminative, diaphoretic, expectorant, and sedative. They provide the immune system with a useful boost if you are suffering from coughs, colds, catarrh, or bronchitis.

- Make an infusion from one to two teaspoons per cup. Or take ¼ to 1 teaspoon of the tincture three times a day.

Peppermint

Peppermint was discussed at the end of the stomach section because of its excellent action as a carminative (p.96). However, it also very useful for the immune system.

As a diaphoretic, it is an excellent remedy for colds and the flu, helping to clear the head and increase the elimination of toxins. The vapor helps to clear blocked sinuses and nasal passages and to relieve associated sinus and congestion headaches. It combines well with boneset, elder, and yarrow for this purpose. Drink it hot, as a tea, for maximum benefit.

Pleurisy Root

Pleurisy root is discussed fully in Chapter 13 on the lungs, for which, as it name implies, it is a beneficial herb (p.181). However, it also merits a mention here, as it is a useful general diaphoretic as well as being a specific herb for the lungs.

Yarrow

Yarrow is discussed in the chapter on your kidneys (p.171). It, too, deserves a mention here, as it is a useful general diaphoretic as well as addressing problems of the urinary tract.

KICK-A-GERM-JOY-JUICE

It is hard to resist this one — even the name gets you in. I learned it in my early days as a naturopath from a colleague, Russell Frank Atkinson. I have somewhat embellished his recipe over the years, but can highly recommend the result if you have a cold or flu, are feeling in need of a good pick-me-up, and if you are tired of lying around feeling ill with a thick head and blocked sinuses and simply want to get well and get on with life.

Combine equal amounts of powdered ginger and garlic, add a bunch of peppermint leaves and a pinch of cayenne pepper. Pour on boiling water, add the juice of one lemon, freshly squeezed, and sweeten to taste with honey. This will liven you up, clear your head, and help to reduce your temperature.

Once the jolt is over, it is time to make a tea from boneset and catnip in combination with either echinacea or cat's claw. In between times, replace your lost fluids with elderberry cordial, and make a salad that includes nasturtium and dandelion leaves with plenty of fresh garlic in the dressing.

No self-respecting cold or flu can stay around for long when faced with this onslaught; and you will have had a good, effective, and thorough cleanout.

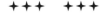

✦ CHAPTER 11 ✦

Your Lymphatic System

ONCE TOXINS HAVE BROKEN your digestive system barrier and entered your bloodstream, they are free to travel throughout your body. The same is true for toxins that are produced internally. We have discussed the role of your immune system in dealing with these toxins. It is now time to discuss the role of your lymphatic system. This system is somewhat analogous to either the street sweeper that cleans your streets and removes the household wastes or to the vacuum cleaner with which you remove the dust from the rooms of your home at regular (or irregular) intervals.

To eliminate toxic wastes, two things have to happen. First, the toxins in your bloodstream have to be eliminated from there, and this is usually done via the kidneys, which filter your blood and transfer the toxins to the urine that will be expelled. However, many toxins will escape from your bloodstream and enter your tissues; others will have been produced in your tissues themselves. So second, these escaped toxins have to be rounded up and either destroyed or returned to the bloodstream so they can be sent to your kidneys.

This is where your lymphatic system comes into play. Your tissues consist of a variety of different types of cells. All these cells contain fluids that can contain toxins. Some of this fluid returns to the bloodstream of its own accord, but not all of it. So there is a second transport system that can help to extract these fluids from your tissues and either deal with the toxins they contain or return them and the fluid to your bloodstream. It's called your lymphatic system.

Your lymphatic system, unlike your bloodstream, is a one-way system. It carries fluids back into your bloodstream. Think of your lymphatic system, if you like, as a multi-tentacled hoovering system that collects up the dispersed fluids and returns them to where they are needed.

However, this is not just a simple process of moving fluids around. At the same time as collecting these fluids, your lymphatics collect up many of the waste products that have been produced by your normal cellular activity. They also collect other debris and toxins including viruses and bacteria. Your lymph, this fluid with its contents, travels along your lymphatic vessels that pass up your arms and legs and up your trunk. On the way, your lymph passes through your lymph glands. These are situated throughout your body but are concentrated in several specific areas, such as at the back of your knees and in your groin, your elbows and armpits, in your trunk at various points along the main blood vessels, and in your neck. It is in these glands that you deal with bacteria and viruses, and it is these glands that swell up and become tender and painful while doing this vital job, when you have a cold or other infection.

Without this lymphatic system, fluids and toxins would build up in your tissues. Eventually the lymphatic fluid enters your veins near your heart and so enters your bloodstream. From here the blood eventually reaches your kidneys and is filtered, the toxins being removed, as before, in your urine.

Individual Herbs to Help Your Lymphatic System

There are a number of herbs that exert a beneficial effect on the lymphatic system and help it do its work better. Obviously these should be considered when you are planning an herbal Detox Regime. They include cleavers, echinacea, golden seal, marigold, and poke root.

Cleavers

Cleavers also goes by the lovely name of goosegrass, the more apt names of grip grass or everlasting friendship, or the Latin name of *Galium aparine*. It can be found growing wild in hedges and ditches and along the sides of roads, and does well in cool climates. You may be familiar with it as the weed that grows through everything, fastening itself ladder-like as it surges toward daylight through even the densest of vegetation. When pulled, it willingly comes away in armfuls.

It should be collected before flowering, with the green parts, stems, and small leaves used. They are alterative, anti-inflammatory, antineoplastic, astringent, diuretic, and tonic.

This means that cleavers offers several benefits when you are Detoxing. It enhances the function of your lymphatic system and is frequently recommended for swollen glands in general and for specific problems such as swollen tonsils. Thus, it improves the ability of your lymphatic system to deal with toxins. For this purpose, it combines and works well with poke root.

As a diuretic, cleavers increases fluid loss and the excretion of urine, again, with its load of toxins. Furthermore, as an anti-inflammatory, it helps in the treatment of cystitis. Cleavers is also a general blood cleanser, so it is useful if there are associated skin problems (see below).

- Make an infusion allowing two to three teaspoons of the dried herb to the cup. If you prefer to use the tincture, take ½ to 1 teaspoon three times a day.

STEAMED CLEAVERS

Cleavers can also be cooked as a green vegetable. Haul it, in armfuls, off whatever vegetation you find it smothering. Use all the green parts, stems and leaves, chop, steam lightly and serve with a dash of olive oil and black pepper. Delicious. My goats love it, too, but then this is not always the best of recommendations.

Golden Seal

Golden seal is another amazingly useful herb and one that we touched on when discussing your stomach (p.93). However, it plays many different roles and is a valuable part of any attempt to clean up your system no matter where the problem is. We could put its detailed discussion in many different sections, but here, where we are talking about your lymphatic system and immune system, is a particularly appropriate place.

Golden seal, or *Hydrastis canadensis*, is an antiinflammatory, antipyretic, antifungal, anticatarrhal, antimalarial, antiparasitic, anodyne, astringent, laxative, muscular stimulant, bitter, oxytocic, and a tonic. It also combines well with other herbs.

One of its most important roles is the result of its effect on the skin and all the mucous membranes. It strengthens and tones them, which leads to its use in a wide variety of situations. As an antifungal, it helps fight *Candida albicans*, one of the most common fungal infections that adversely affects many thousands of woman. *Candida albicans* damages the lining not only of the digestive tract but also of the genito-urinary tract. Because of its action on mucous membranes and because it is useful against a number of micro-organisms, it can be used beneficially as a douche for vaginitis. It can also be used as a cream. It is used for excessive menstrual bleeding, menstrual irregularities, during labor and for prostatitis.

Because of its actions against a number of infectious agents, it is useful in supporting the immune system against bacterial and fungal infections. When this is combined with its action on mucous membranes, it is obviously a useful herb for conditions such as catarrh, upper respiratory tract infections, colds, flu, glandular swelling and fever, so we will talk about it again when we discuss your lungs.

Finally, it helps a number of skin conditions including eczema, pruritis, and ringworm; and can be used externally as a wash for cuts, abrasions and skin infections, and in the treatment of conjunctivitis. So we will discuss it again there, too.

One word of warning: because of its oxytocic action, it should not be taken during pregnancy without professional advice until labor commences.

- For an infusion, allow ½ to 1 teaspoonful of the dried herb per cup. This can be drunk, and it can also be used externally as a wash. If you prefer the tincture, take ½ to 1 teaspoon three times a day, or it can be used externally as a cream

Poke Root

Poke root, or *Phytolacca americana*, is another herb that is particularly helpful for the lymphatic system. As its name implies, it is the root that is used, and it should be dug up either in late autumn or in spring. It is anticatarrhal, antirheumatic, emetic, purgative, and a stimulant.

We will discuss it later, as it can contribute to a Detox Regime by way of its effect on the respiratory system (p.182) and on the skin (p.188), but for the moment, our focus is on the lymphatic drainage system. Here, poke root is used in the treatment of adenitis, tonsillitis, and laryngitis. It is an excellent herb to use if there are swollen glands in any part of the body. It has been used in the treatment of mumps, mastitis (as an external poultice), and fibrocystic breast disease.

When treating problems related to the lymphatic system, it combines well with blue flag.

- For a decoction, use ⅓ teaspoon per cup, simmered for 15 minutes. For a tincture, use ⅛ to ¼ teaspoon three times a day. Care should be taken not to increase this dose, as it can then become quite a strong laxative

Wild Indigo Root

The root of wild indigo, or *Baptisia tinctoria,* should be dug up in the autumn after flowering has stopped, cleaned, cut up, and dried thoroughly. It is an antimicrobial, anticatarrhal, and febrifuge.

It is an excellent herb for cleaning up the lymphatic system or dealing with an excessive production of catarrh, be it white and clear or yellow and infected. In fact, it is an excellent herb for any problem where there is a particular site of infection. If you have mouth ulcers or gingivitis, or inflammation of the gums, wild indigo root can be used as a mouthwash. If you have pyorrhoea, when there is infection or inflammation of the bones of your jaw and around your teeth, possibly with erosions of the bones and loosening of the teeth, but certainly with infection, use wild indigo root first as a mouthwash and then swallow the tincture for its systemic benefit in fighting the infection.

Wild indigo is useful if there is excessive mucus production. This may be caused by food allergies or by either an excessive intake of dairy products or even an acute reaction to the intake of any dairy products at all. In these instances, the offending foods should be avoided. While these corrections are being made, and to assist in returning the tissues to normal, wild indigo root can be used.

The root can also be used for any catarrhal infections of the nose or sinuses; for infections of the ears, nose, or throat; or for laryngitis, pharyngitis, or tonsillitis. Use it if your lymph glands are swollen or if you have a temperature. Its benefits don't stop there. It can be used as a douche for vaginitis or thrush.

In the treatment of infections, you can combine it with echinacea and myrrh; and for lymphatic problems, with cleavers and poke root.

- For a decoction, use ⅓ teaspoon per cup, simmered for 15 minutes, and drink this three times a day. Alternatively, take ¼ to ½ teaspoon of the tincture three times a day.

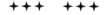

✦ Chapter 12 ✦

Your Kidneys and Bladder

A DISCUSSION OF YOUR LYMPHATIC SYSTEM leads naturally to a discussion of your kidneys as an excretory route for toxins.

We have already discovered that many substances are excreted from your body in fecal matter. Much of this fecal matter is unabsorbed food, fiber and microorganisms, but it includes a variety of mainly fat-soluble toxins secreted from your body via your liver and bile duct. As you have already discovered, your liver has a vast range of jobs to perform. In addition to excreting mainly fat-soluble toxins via your bile duct, it also processes a lot of them and changes them into a water-soluble form so that they can then be excreted, via your kidneys, in your urine.

Your kidneys have a more focused role. Dominantly, their job is two-fold, that of maintaining various proper balances and that of excretion. A third role is the production of a hormone called rennin that is involved in maintaining normal blood pressure so your kidneys can filter properly.

Your Kidneys and Excretion

Your kidneys cannot simply excrete everything that comes their way. They have to be selective, and they do this via a two-step process. First, they let most substances enter the urine, then they filter it and reabsorb the many compounds that are needed. These include such compounds as glucose, amino acids, and minerals that were circulating in the bloodstream. These useful substances cannot be allowed to simply drain out of the body in the urine. Many systemic toxins, those made within your body, are excreted via the kidneys, as are most of the water-soluble toxins that you have taken in.

Your Kidneys As Balancers

Your kidneys perform a number of balancing roles. They help to balance the amount of fluid in your body. If you drink more, you urinate more; if you drink less, you urinate less. It is your kidneys that monitor this situation and ensure that you do not become either dehydrated or overhydrated.

Your kidneys also monitor your salt levels. In Stone Age times, salt, or specifically sodium, was scarce. Potassium was found in relative abundance in all the plant foods that were available. The kidneys therefore developed the capacity to hold on to sodium and prevent its loss, while allowing the excess potassium to leave in the urine.

This presents the kidneys with a problem today since people eat relatively small amounts of vegetables and get relatively little potassium in their diet, while at the same time eating large amounts of salt. Your kidneys have not kept up with this social and dietary development, allowing the now relatively rare potassium to flow away freely while still hanging on to and retaining the over-abundant sodium. The amount of sodium in your diet is a strain on your kidneys and makes its work of maintaining a proper mineral balance and a proper fluid balance all the more difficult.

You often hear about the acid or alkaline balance in your body. It is important not to be either too acidic or too alkaline. Because of our present diet, it is more common for people to be too acidic. Achieving the proper balance between these states is yet another job for your kidneys, albeit one that it does in conjunction with your lungs.

Your Kidneys and the Hormone Rennin

For your kidneys to do their filtering job properly, there needs to be sufficient pressure on the blood flow entering the kidneys. To ensure that this is the case, your kidneys are able to produce the hormone rennin, which can raise blood pressure. This means that if, for instance, your arteries are partly blocked and the local blood pressure is reduced, then your kidneys will increase their output of rennin and raise the blood pressure to a point where efficient filtering can occur. Unfortunately for you, rennin is not selective, and it will increase the blood pressure throughout your body. That is a problem, but does not concern the kidneys, which are focusing on their own specific needs.

This means that a real part of any Detox program should be to keep your arteries clear so your kidneys can do their job properly without increasing your blood pressure — but that is a whole other story and one we do not have room for here.

Your Kidneys and Detox

Clearly it is vital for a good Detox Regime that your kidneys are working to their very best ability. Adequate fluid intake is essential for the proper functioning of your kidneys, and the role of water in any cleansing program is vital. An adequate fluid intake is also important so that you can avoid and get rid of any problems such as cystitis or thrush.

A diet rich in a wide variety of nutrient-rich vegetables and fruits will benefit your kidneys, and there are also many herbs that can be of assistance.

Diuretic Herbs

Diuretic herbs are those that increase the flow of urine. In general, they will not lead to dehydration, but they will help to avoid problems of excessive fluid retention. At the same time, by normalizing urine flow, they will help to encourage the elimination of toxins. You should drink plenty of water while you are taking them to increase the flushing effect of the kidneys and thus aid detoxification.

Dandelion

We discussed dandelion when we discussed the role of your liver (p.125). It is an excellent liver herb, particularly the root. It is also an excellent kidney herb, and for this purpose, you can use the root or the leaves. It is almost impossible to drink a cup of dandelion coffee (from the root) or dandelion tea (from the leaves) without noticing a need to urinate soon afterwards. Unlike other diuretics, it offers the additional advantage that it is rich in potassium, and as we have seen, this is a mineral that is readily lost via the kidneys and needs to be replaced when a diuretic is taken. Keep in mind that the amount of potassium in your diet can be increased by eating more fruit and vegetables, which should feature prominently in any Detox Regime.

When you are using this as a kidney herb and diuretic, it combines well with couchgrass, corn silk, buchu, and yarrow.

Cleavers

Cleavers was discussed under the lymphatic system where it exerts its major benefits. However, it is also a valuable diuretic. This means that in addition to helping to drain toxins and excess fluid from your tissues and deliver them back to the bloodstream, it helps the kidneys to process both these toxins and waste fluids.

Boldo

Boldo was also discussed when we considered the role of the liver (p.133). However, it too is a useful diuretic and antiseptic and can be helpful in cases of cystitis as well as when you need a diuretic. Because of its demulcent character, it can also help to soothe and heal the mucous membranes lining the bladder and urethra, particularly if there has been any local damage or inflammation.

Buchu

The leaves of buchu, or *Agathosma betulina* (*Rutacea*), should be collected while the plant is flowering and fruiting, and is a diuretic and urinary antiseptic.

Buchu is virtually a specific for the kidneys. It increases the flow of urine and acts as an antiseptic in the treatment of cystitis, urethritis, and prostatitis, burning and painful urination, and related problems. In cystitis and other situations that involve sensations of pain or burning on urination, it combines well with couch grass, marsh mallow, and yarrow.

- Make the infusion allowing 1 or 2 teaspoons of the leaves per cup, and drink this three times a day; or take ½ to 1 teaspoon of the tincture three times a day.

Couch Grass

It is the rhizome of couch grass, or *Agropyron repens,* that is used in herbal medicine. It is dug up in either spring or early autumn and acts as a diuretic, demulcent, and antimicrobial. For these reasons, it is particularly useful for any problems of the urinary system ranging from cystitis, urethritis, prostatitis, and prostatic hypertrophy, to kidney stones and gravel. As a diuretic, it offers the additional benefit of being rich in potassium. In fact, you should really take a range of minerals, as it is not just potassium that is lost when you urinate. Fortunately, herbs do, in general, contain a range of trace minerals.

Couch grass combines well with buchu and yarrow for urinary tract infections, and with hydrangea for prostate problems

- It is best made as a decoction for which you should allow 2 teaspoons per cup; or, take 1 to 1½ teaspoon of tincture twice a day.

Urinary Antiseptics

If your system is toxic or you have picked up infections, the urinary tract is a likely target. You may have a fungal infection such as vaginal thrush, with its discharge and localized vaginal itch and discomfort. You may get repeated bouts of cystitis or inflammation of the bladder, which leads to a frequent and overwhelmingly urgent need to urinate, even when there is very little urine there to pass, plus localized burning and pain. Or the infection may be further up, even in the kidneys.

It is difficult for the proper elimination of toxins to take place if your kidneys are infected, so herbs that can help treat any local infection in them will be helpful. If the problems relate to thrush or cystitis, then these symptoms have to be resolved themselves as part of your cleansing program.

Bearberry

Bearberry, or *Arctostaphylos uva-ursi,* is an herb that is often better known by its second or Latin name, *Uva ursi.* This is the name homeopaths use for it, and it is a very important remedy for many different problems of the urinary tract. The leaves should be collected in spring or summer.

Bearberry is astringent, antiseptic, demulcent, and diuretic, and exerts these activities most convincingly in the urinary tract and acts on the mucous membranes there. It is useful for kidney infections, kidney stones, and gravel. It is useful as an antiseptic in the treatment of cystitis. By its demulcent and healing action on the mucous membranes, it is helpful in the treatment of thrush. In addition, it has been used successfully in the treatment of bed-wetting, possibly aided by its astringent action, whereby it tightens up the tissues.

For the treatment of cystitis, it combines well with corn silk, couch grass, and yarrow.

A word of warning. It has a mild oxytocic effect, and though it is only mild, it is best not to use this herb during pregnancy, although it can be used, often with great benefit, once labor has started.

It can be used externally, as a douche, in the treatment of vaginitis, thrush, or infections or ulcerations of the vagina.

- Make the infusion from 1 to 2 teaspoons of the herb in a cup of boiling water, or take ½ to 1 teaspoon of the tincture three times a day.

Birch

Birch, or more specifically, silver birch, goes by the Latin name of *Betula pendula (Betulaceae).* Its wonderful silvery-white bark is distinctive and gives a glade of these trees a light and shimmering quality. It grows well in many situations, but particularly well on wet and acid soil.

The leaves and bark are used. Young leaves should be collected in spring and early summer. When collecting the bark, be careful to collect it from only one side of the tree. Do not make a cut that goes the whole way around the trunk at any point, or the tree, like any other that is ringbarked in the same way, will die.

It is an excellent antiseptic for the urinary tract, helping in the treatment of cystitis and other related infections, and for this purpose can be combined with bearberry. However, it is also useful in situations where there is fluid retention in general, and in particular it is useful in the treatment of rheumatism and arthritis. It is thought that this latter effect could be due to the cleansing effect, the removal of toxins from the affected tissues.

An interesting use for the bark exists. If you are ever out walking among silver birch trees and sprain or strain a muscle, strip off a small patch of the bark and apply the inside — damp, if possible — to the affected muscle. It is said to help to relieve the strain. Again, however, do be careful not to ringbark the tree.

As a tincture, in the treatment of rheumatism, it combines well with black willow.

- Make an infusion from 1 to 2 teaspoons of the dried leaves and allow them to infuse for ten minutes. The tincture dose is Ω¼ to ½ teaspoon three times a day.

Celery Seed

Celery is familiar to most people as a vegetable. It hardly even needs identifying by its Latin name, but for the sake of completeness we will do so — it is *Apium graveolens*. The vegetable is good for you — it's an excellent source of very obvious fiber for one thing — but the seed is also beneficial. The plant needs to flower and the fruit needs to be allowed to ripen. Then in the autumn, the seed can be collected. For most people, however, a quick trip to the grocery shelves will produce a jar of celery seeds.

The seeds are antirheumatic, carminative, diuretic, and sedative. The main medicinal use of celery seed, traditionally, is in the treatment of arthritis, rheumatism, and gout; and for the latter it works well with bogbean. However, it is also a useful diuretic, not perhaps one that we would focus on primarily, but it works well with dandelion and is such a useful culinary herb that it is worth considering. Add celery seeds to your diet, to salad dressings, and in cooking whenever the flavor appeals to you, sure in the knowledge that it is also contributing to your Detox Regime.

- Or, you can make an infusion allowing 1 to 2 teaspoons of the seeds per cup; or take the tincture, ½ to 1 teaspoon, three times a day.

DIURETIC SALAD WITH DRESSING

Potassium-rich vegetables will help your body to maintain its correct sodium-potassium balance and help you to prevent or treat fluid retention.

For the salad:
Select the leaves of cleavers, dandelion, elder, greater celandine, pansy, and 1 bunch celery; remove the tough outer stems and chop finely. Keep the leaves separate, but chop them, too.
a bunch of watercress
1 endive
a wedge of watermelon — remove the skin and seeds, dice the flesh
1 cucumber, diced (there is no need to remove the skin unless it is not organic)
a bunch of fresh asparagus spears, lightly steamed

Combine the cubes of cucumber and water melon, and build a ring around the edge of a flat platter. Combine the chopped leaves of your chosen herbs, chopped celery stems, chopped endive, and the watercress and spread over the center of the platter. Lay the asparagus spears on top, and sprinkle over a handful of fresh chervil, parsley, and tarragon leaves.

For the dressing:
Combine three parts of virgin olive oil with one part of wine vinegar. Then add as much and as many of the following herbs as you like: celery seed, golden rod (sometimes

---

available, dried, as Solidago tea), crushed juniper berries, and a pinch of mustard powder. Combine all ingredients and drizzle over the salad. Decorate with a few borage or daisy petals.

Juniper

Juniperus communis is a small shrub, and it is the berries that are used in herbal medicine. These are the same berries that give gin its distinctive flavor. They should be collected in the autumn when they are ripe.

Juniper is generally thought of as an herb for the urinary tract, where it is an excellent antiseptics, and diuretic, frequently used in the treatment of cystitis and prostatisis. For problems involving the kidneys themselves, there are better herbs you can choose.

In addition, juniper has other beneficial actions. It is an antirheumatic, so it is particularly useful if, as well as wanting to go on a cleansing program, you also have to deal with arthritis or rheumatism, or even simply generalized pain in the muscles and joints.

Last, it is a carminative and can be used in the treatment of colic and flatulence until you get your digestion under control. This should be considered as a beneficial additional activity of this herb, useful if you have digestive as well as urinary tract problems, not as a prime reason for selecting juniper.

It is best not to use this herb during pregnancy.

- For the infusion, allow one teaspoon of the crushed berries per cup, and drink this night and morning.

Yarrow

Yarrow, or *Achillea millefolium*, is a delicate plant, and everything that grows above ground is used to make the herbal remedy. It should be gathered between June and September and is a diaphoretic, hypotensive, astringent, diuretic, and antiseptic, and is of particular use to the immune system. It can help to relieve a fever without suppressing it so that you get the benefit of the raised temperature. This facilitates your immune system and encourages the excretion of toxins, without the fever having to become too severe.

In the urinary tract, it is particularly useful in the treatment of cystitis, and for this purpose, combines well with bearberry, corn silk and couch grass.

- For the infusion allow 1 to 2 teaspoons per cup, or take ½ to 1 teaspoon of the tincture three times a day.

+++ +++

✦ CHAPTER 13 ✦

Your Lungs

YOUR BOWELS AND YOUR KIDNEYS obviously play a major role in the elimination of waste products and toxins from your body. However, your lungs are also important. They play a smaller though still significant role in elimination.

First, it is via your lungs that you get rid of most of the carbon dioxide you produce. When you eat food for energy, a number of reactions take place. After the food has been digested, the various components — glucose from the starches, fruits, vegetables and sugars, plus the fats — are absorbed into your bloodstream and carried to the various cells in your body. These cells then take up the glucose or fats they need for energy. To produce energy these fats and the glucose are combined with the oxygen that you breathe in and converted into carbon dioxide and water. Most of the water is released in your urine. Most of the carbon dioxide leaves in the exhaled air from your lungs as you breathe out. This is part of your elimination procedure. It is also via this process that your lungs help your kidneys to maintain your body's correct acid-alkaline balance.

There are other things happening in and around your lungs that have an important bearing on Detoxing. When you breathe in, you are drawing into your lungs not only air with its all important oxygen, but also the toxins that it contains, be they gases, particulate matter, or microorganisms. To help to block the uptake of the particulate matter and microorganisms, the cells that line your bronchial tubes have tiny hairlike structures. They can bend and curl in only one direction, rather like the fingers on your hand. They protrude into the space of your bronchial tubes and straighten out as you breathe in. In this way, they lie across the hollow tube and are able to act as filters. When you breathe out, the structures bend, like your fingers, curling upwards, and thus act as sweepers, propelling the particles back up the tubes, on your exhaled breath, on their way back to your nose or mouth. Their job is made easier by the production of a normal and healthy amount of mucus. This mucus sticks to the particles and prevents you breathing them in further. It also encourages the expulsion of the unwanted visitors as you are stimulated to cough and or blow them out.

Thus, some mucus *is* beneficial. It is only the excessive production of unwanted mucus that is to be avoided. Some foods, particularly in susceptible people, are likely to trigger this excessive mucus production. The foods most commonly implicated are dairy products, usually cow's milk and its products, but possibly also goat, sheep, and other types of milks and their products. The second most likely group of culprits are the grains. Wheat is the most likely of these to trigger excess mucus production, followed by barley, oats and rye, but all of the grains, including spelt, corn, millet, rice, quinoa and others can do the same thing in susceptible people.

These mucus-forming foods may not even show up in allergy testing in affected people. It is possible that the only symptom they produce is the production of mucus. However, it is also possible that they may indeed be systemic allergens as well for the person concerned, and may be causing other, unrecognized, problems. Alternatively, there may be other foods that the person is allergic to, and one of the symptoms these allergens cause may be the production of the excess mucus. To summarize, mucus production can be caused by dairy products or grains, whether or not they are allergens, and by all substances to which the individual is allergic.

While, in the following section, we are considering detoxification in total, we will also have to deal with a range of catarrhal problems including colds, influenza, bronchitis, and related problems. It is essential that you have totally healthy lungs and bronchial tubes if you want to be fully healthy and avoid the build-up of toxins.

Expectorants

Herbs that help you to expel mucus and other unwanted material from your lungs are called expectorants. These are useful if you suffer from an excessive production of mucus, from catarrh, from phlegm in the back of your nose and throat, or from postnasal drip.

If you simply *have* to have a handkerchief with you at all times, or if you never seem to have a clear head or clear sinuses, these expectorants could be just the herbs you need.

However, it is worth reminding you that you could be suffering from allergies, either food allergies or environmental allergies, possibly from both. However good the herbs are and however appropriate your choice, if allergic reactions continue and keep causing the problem, you will not be able to solve the situation unless you eliminate the cause. So consider having some allergy tests done as well as taking expectorant herbs.

Coltsfoot

The Latin name for coltsfoot, *Tussilago farfara*, is more evocative of its purpose than its common name, since *tussis* is another word for cough and *tussive* means "about or pertaining to a cough." This is an excellent herb for clearing out the lungs and bronchial tubes.

The flowers should be collected before they are in full bloom, so in practice this means collecting them in the spring. The leaves can be collected in early summer. They are frequently used in combination remedies; and their action is anticatarrhal, antitussive, demulcent, diuretic, and expectorant. This means that they can offer many benefits to a Detox Regime, as they work on many different parts of the body.

Coltsfoot is known mainly as a lung herb and is helpful in cases ranging from irritable coughs and phlegm to more severe lung problems such as bronchitis, asthma, whooping cough, and emphysema. It combines well with horehound and comfrey, two other herbs that are covered in this section.

It is also useful in the treatment of cystitis, but this is a lesser use. It does mean, however, that if you have both problems, this is a particularly useful herb.

We have yet to talk about your skin as an organ of elimination, but it is worth pointing out here that coltsfoot can also help in the treatment of boils, abscesses, bedsores, and ulcers. In these instances, it is best used as a poultice.

- For the infusion, use one to two teaspoons per cup. For the tincture, take ½ to 1 teaspoon three times a day.

Comfrey

Comfrey is a well-known herb. Its large, furry leaves, often over a foot long, spring up in abundance each spring, then die down again in autumn until only the tiniest sign of the plant remains above ground, while the underground roots multiply. It is beloved by gardeners, particularly organic gardeners. It can be used in trenches as a fertilizer or made into liquid manure. This latter is made by filling a barrel with the leaves, filling this up with water, and then, a few weeks later, using this liquid to fertilize the soil around your vegetables and flowers. It is also sought after by many animals, including my goats who will break down fences to get to it.

Its Latin name, and the name homoeopaths use for it, is *Symphytum officinale,* and its family name *Boraginaceae* alerts you to the fact that it is in the same family as borage, another herb with a furry leaf that pops up year after year no matter what you might do to erase it. This is no bad thing, as borage is also an expectorant as well as being a diaphoretic anti-inflammatory, tonic, and galactogogue. Its blue flowers make a colorful addition to a salad, but I digress.

The leaves of comfrey can be gathered at any time; the roots and rhizomes should be dug up in spring and autumn. The herb acts as an astringent, demulcent, expectorant, and vulnerary.

Like coltsfoot, comfrey is helpful in the treatment of irritable coughs and productive bronchitis and helps to loosen mucus, both clear and infected, from your system. However, the best results come when you use the two herbs in combination.

Comfrey offers further benefits, this time to your digestive system. It is helpful in the treatment of damaged mucosa. This means it can be helpful if you have a hiatus hernia, stomach or duodenal ulcer, inflammation of the small or large intestine, or ulcerative colitis. For these problems, it works particularly well when combined with slippery elm powder (p.105) and aloe vera juice.

Comfrey will also be mentioned later in regard to your skin (p.195), as it is an excellent herb for many skin problems.

- To make the infusion, allow 1 to 3 teaspoons of the finely chopped herb per cup, or take ½ to 1 teaspoon of the tincture three times a day.

Daisy

The common lawn daisy is either a delight to the eye for the romantic, or a perennial problem for those who love a smooth green lawn. Few people think of it as a beneficial herb. Yet daisy, or *Bellis perennis*, is an excellent herb for our present purposes and one that is readily available. All you need to do, all summer long, is go outside and collect it. In fact, it can be collected from spring to autumn, throughout its growing season. Collect the flowerheads, not the leaves, and either dry them or use them fresh. Daisy is an expectorant and astringent.

This is another herb that, like comfrey, combines well with coltsfoot. It can also be used with golden rod. Its astringent action allows it to help if your cleansing is going too fast and you have diarrhea. It also helps in conditions such as rheumatism and arthritis, and for liver or kidney problems.

- Make a tea, using one teaspoon of the dried flower heads per cup, and drink this three or four times a day to help eliminate catarrh or soothe a cough. If you prefer the tincture, take ½ to 1 teaspoon three times a day.

Elecampane

Elecampane, or *Inula helenium*, is, like the daisy, in the *Compositae* family. However, this time it is the rhizome that is used. It should be dug up in the autumn and is an antibacterial, antitussive expectorant and stomachic.

Its major use is for problems of the respiratory system where it can be used if there is a bacterial infection. If you have a temperature, it will help to reduce this gradually and productively by maximizing the excretion of toxins in the perspiration, so the temperature can do its job for you without being excessive. It is used for tickling productive coughs and bronchitis and will help to clear out unwanted mucus and toxins. It is helpful in more serious lung problems such as emphysema, asthma, bronchial asthma, and tuberculosis.

It is a good herb to choose if you also have a sluggish digestive system, as it helps to stimulate the latter.

- For the infusion allow one teaspoon of the herb per cup; for the tincture the dosage is one to two mls three times a day.

Grindelia

Grindelia camporum is yet another herb in the daisy family that is useful for catarrhal problems associated with the lungs. The parts of the herb above the ground are used and should be collected before the flower buds open, and dried as soon as possible. Grindelia is an antispasmodic, expectorant, and hypotensive.

As an expectorant, it helps to get rid of catarrh from the upper respiratory tract. It relaxes the muscles of the lungs and bronchial tubes and helps with bronchial problems and asthma. Contrary to popular belief, the difficulty for asthmatics is not in breathing *in,* it is in relaxing the bronchial muscles and being able to breathe *out,* to get rid of the old air so there is space to take in the new. So, relaxing herbs are helpful, particularly useful in asthma and other lung problems when they are associated with an increased heartbeat or nervous tension such as nervous asthma. Grindelia can also be used in the treatment of whooping cough. It works well in these conditions when combined with lobelia and pill-bearing spurge.

Going further with respect to these comments about the heart, you can use this herb when you also have high blood pressure, as it helps to relax the smooth muscles of the arteries and the heart muscle itself.

- For the infusion, allow 1 teaspoon of the herb per cup, infuse for 10 to 15 minutes, and drink three times a day; or take ¼ to ½ teaspoon of the tincture three times a day.

Horehound

Use the dried leaves and flowers of horehound or *Marrubium vulgare*. These should be collected while the plant is in blossom, usually between June to September, and dried at a moderate temperature (below 95°F). It, is an expectorant, antispasmodic, bitter digestive, and vulnerary.

This means that it can help in detoxification in several ways.

It acts on the lungs and relaxes the muscles while also encouraging mucus production and clearing. As an antispasmodic, it can be used for bronchial spasms and for nonproductive coughs, as well as productive coughs. Use it in combination with coltsfoot, mullein, and lobelia to help clear out your lungs.

It will also help cleansing via the digestive system by stimulating the flow of bile and encouraging normal elimination.

As a vulnerary, it can be applied externally to open wounds, where it will encourage rapid healing.

- For the infusion, allow up to 1 teaspoon of the herb per cup, or take ¼ to ½ teaspoon of the tincture three times a day.

Lobelia

The above-ground parts of *Lobelia inflata* should be collected after the plant has flowered, from late summer to early autumn.

Lobelia is one of the best known and most effective herbs for the treatment of lung problems, from minor coughs and infections to deep-seated bronchial asthma and heavy and sticky phlegm. It is an antiasthmatic, antispasmodic, expectorant, respiratory stimulant, and emetic. It is often found in a range of products designed to help eliminate catarrh, deal with coughs, and clear the lungs, and is recommended for the treatment of asthma as well as bronchial and congestive problems. It is a strong-acting herb and should be used with caution.

- Infuse ¼ to ½ of a teaspoon of the herb per cup, or take ⅛ to ¼ teaspoon of the tincture three times a day.

Linseed

Linseed has been discussed under the digestive system. It is also a useful lung herb. As a demulcent, antitussive, and emollient, it can help clear your lungs. It has been used in the treatment of irritating coughs and lung infections such as bronchitis. It can also be used externally as a chest poultice for the treatment of pleurisy and other lung problems.

So if you are constipated *and* have lung problems, be sure to use linseed instead of psyllium hulls to get your bowels moving, and your lungs will benefit as well.

Lungwort

Both its general name and its Latin name *Pulmonaria officinalis* indicate the fact that this is a valuable herb for lung problems. The leaves are used and can be collected from spring to autumn.

As an astringent, it helps in the treatment of diarrhea and hemorrhoids, and it can be used externally to tighten the tissues and promote healing of cuts.

However, its main and most important use is definitely for the respiratory system. Lungwort is a demulcent, expectorant, astringent, and vulnerary, and it is the first two actions that particularly concern us. It helps to clear catarrh from the upper respiratory tract, from the nose and throat to the upper bronchial tubes, and is used in the treatment of coughs and bronchitis. Use it in combination with coltsfoot, lobelia, and horehound.

- For the infusion, allow one to two teaspoons per cup. The tincture dose can be from ¼ to 1 teaspoon three times a day.

Mullein

Mullein, or *Verbascum thapsus,* is another herb whose area of application is dominantly the respiratory system but which has several benefits to offer in a Detox Regime. Collect the leaves in midsummer and the flowers in late summer. They are demulcent, expectorant, and vulnerary, mildly diuretic, and sedative.

As a demulcent, mullein is soothing to the mucous membranes and helps to reduce local inflammation and pain. This includes the internal lining of your nose, throat, and bronchial tubes, and also those of your digestive system. As a diuretic, albeit a mild one, it will help to encourage the elimination of toxins in your urine, and it can be used externally as a soothing poultice on areas of inflammation or to encourage healing.

However, it is particularly valuable if you are trying to clear out your respiratory tract and is used in the treatment of hard dry coughs, sore throats, and bronchitis.

- Make an infusion from one to two teaspoons of the herb per cup, or take ¼ to 1 teaspoon of the tincture three times a day.

Pleurisy Root

Pleurisy root, or *Aesclepias tuberosa,* is particularly useful if you have a lot of unwanted catarrh or mucus. As the name implies, it is the root, or more accurately, the rhizome, that is used. It should be dug up in spring, and is an antispasmodic, carminative, diuretic, and expectorant.

It was described in the section on the lymphatic system (p.155), but is also a very valuable herb for the lungs. If you are producing a lot of mucus or troubled with catarrh, then take this herb combined with coltsfoot. For asthma and other more deep-seated lung problems, it combines well with lobelia.

- Make an infusion allowing ½ to 1 teaspoon per cup, or take ¼ to ½ teaspoon of the tincture three times a day.

Red Clover

Trifolium pratense (Papilionaceae) is an excellent herb for any Detox Regime and is discussed in more detail in the section on the skin (p.188), since it is an excellent blood cleanser. However, it is also an excellent expectorant and combines well with many other lung herbs to help get rid of mucus and catarrh.

Thuja

Thuja occidentalis is an evergreen in the conifer family. It is the new green twigs that are used, and these should be collected during the summer to get the best results. Thuja is an astringent, alterative, diuretic, expectorant, and smooth muscle stimulant, although its main benefits derive from its alterative action and its effect on smooth muscles.

In your respiratory system, it is an excellent expectorant for use for bronchial catarrh and is useful in the treatment of coughs, especially if they are dry, irritable coughs or when coughing has become overstimulated and is prolonged.

It is useful in the treatment of such skin conditions as warts, psoriasis, and ringworm. And if vaginal thrush is part of the problem, it can help treat this.

In addition to its role in Detox, it can stimulate a weak heart, help to reduce incontinence, bring on delayed menstruation, assist in the treatment of rheumatism, and reduce the side effects of vaccinations. Altogether, thuja is a very useful herb. Because of its effect on menstruation, it is best not to take this herb during pregnancy as it may provide unwanted stimulation to the uterus.

- For the infusion, use one teaspoon of the herb per cup of boiling water, or take ¼ to ½ teaspoon of the tincture three times a day.

Poke Root

Poke root was discussed under the lymphatic system (p.161) but deserves an extra mention here, as it is helpful in the treatment of catarrh and general respiratory infections.

✛✛✛   ✛✛✛

✦ Chapter 14 ✦

Your Skin

Your skin performs many roles. It does not "hold your body together," or "stop you innards from falling out." On the contrary, it is the forces within your body that hold your skin to your flesh.

Perhaps the most obvious role it offers is protection for the rest of your body from the outside world. By and large, it keeps unwanted substances and organisms out and keeps desirable substances in. It protects your inner organs from light and, to a significant extent, from damage. Thus, it protects your body from the outside world. It also helps you to maintain a constant body temperature. Furthermore, from my point of view, it can be helpful when you are trying to go on a cleansing regime.

Your skin is another organ of elimination. You will be aware that, when exercising or overheated, you sweat, and that when you sweat, salts are also eliminated. Other substances can also be eliminated in this way. Ideally your skin should be minimally involved in toxin elimination; however, it will truly come into play when there is an increase of toxins in the system, and this is often seen in the form of skin problems such as acne, blackheads, white-heads, boils, and cysts. Toxicity is not the only cause of these problems, but can certainly be a contributing factor. Other types of skin problems such as eczema and dermatitis can be caused by allergens, but here, too, toxins may play their part, particularly if allergens are regarded as personal toxins.

Your skin can also be an indicator of general health. Poor skin tone and color and a variety of skin problems as indicated above may indicate deeper health problems. Premature aging of the skin can be a sign that there is premature aging elsewhere and these signs would merit your attention.

There are many types of herbs that can benefit your skin, and which often offer a range of other benefits as well. First, there are the alteratives. These are the herbs that help to clean the blood. They help to cleanse the whole body, and they are particularly useful when the signs of toxicity are seen on the skin. These signs may range from a gray and muddy color to your skin to blackheads, boils, pimples, and cysts.

Blood Cleansers — the Alteratives

Blue Flag

The rhizome of the very beautiful blue flag, or *Iris versicolor* of the *Iridaceae* family should be collected in the autumn. It is anti-inflammatory, alterative, cholagogue, diuretic, and laxative.

It was discussed in the section on your liver (p.133), but its main use is as an alterative for skin problems such as acne, eczema, and psoriasis. As an alterative, its action in these conditions is through cleansing or detoxing the blood. In addition, as a diuretic, it helps to get rid of toxins in the increased flow of urine; as a cholagogue, it encourages proper liver and bile function; and as a gentle laxative, it increases elimination through the bowels. Altogether, this is a good herb offering at least four significant benefits in a Detox Regime.

For our purposes here, it combines well with burdock and yellow dock.

- Infuse ½ to 1 teaspoon of the dried herb per cup of boiling water, or take ½ to 1 teaspoon of the tincture three times a day.

Burdock

Burdock, or *Arctium lappa* of the *Compositae* family is an excellent alterative, or blood cleanser. The roots and rhizome should be dug up in autumn. It is used in such skin conditions such as dry and flaky skin, dandruff, eczema, and in the healing of wounds and ulcers. It is useful in the treatment of psoriasis — whether on its own or associated with arthritis (psoriatic arthritis) or rheumatism (psoriatic rheumatism).

As well as being an alternative it is a diuretic and bitter herb.

This means that it helps to improve digestion by improving stomach function and increasing the secretion of bile. It also helps to increase urinary loss of waste water as well as cleansing the blood, thus helping the skin.

It combines well with red clover or poke root.

- For a decoction allow one teaspoon of the root per cup and simmer for ten minutes. If taking the tincture, take ½ to 1 teaspoon three times a day. As burdock can interfere with iron absorption, it should be taken at a different time of day from any iron supplements.

Cleavers

Cleavers was discussed under the lymphatic system (p.158). As well as helping the lymphatics to clear toxins from your body, it is an excellent blood cleanser and also useful for skin problems. Typically you would use this herb if you have both skin problems and a tendency to swollen get glands or related infections.

Figwort

Figwort has the somewhat unfortunate Latin name of *Scrophularia nodosa* and comes from the *Scrophulariaceae* family. All parts of the plant that grow above ground are used and are collected in summer, while flowering.

It is an alterative, diuretic, cardiac stimulant, and mild laxative. It is useful in the treatment of general heart weakness, although it should not be used if there is tachycardia or a rapid pulse.

It is best known, though, as an herb that is helpful in the treatment of dermatitis, eczema, psoriasis, and any other type of skin irritation. This is added to by its mild laxative effect, which helps to clean the bowels and thus prevent the formation and absorption of toxins in and from that source.

- When making an infusion, allow one to three teaspoons of the fresh herb per cup. The tincture dose is ½ to 1 teaspoon three times a day.

Fumitory

Collect the leaves and flowers of *Fumaria officinalis*, from the *Fumariaceae* family, during summer when the plant is in flower. It is alterative, diuretic, and laxative.

Fumitory thus has all the attributes you could ask of an herb to deal with skin problems in a Detox Regime. It increases the loss of toxins via the stool, urine, and by cleansing the blood, and is used in the treatment of skin problems such as acne and eczema. It combines well with burdock, cleavers, and figwort. It can also be used externally as an eye wash in the treatment of conjunctivitis.

- To make one cup of infusion, use one to two teaspoons of the dried herb and infuse for 10 to 15 minutes. Drink this three times a day, or take ¼ to ½ teaspoon of the tincture three times a day.

Golden Seal

Golden Seal has already been discussed for its role in the digestive system, particularly the stomach (p.93) and colon (p.110), and for its use in improving the function of your lymphatic system (p.159). It can also help your skin.

As, among other things, an anti-inflammatory, antifungal, antiparasitic, astringent agent, it has been used internally in the treatment of eczema, pruritis, ringworm, and externally as a wash for cuts, abrasions, skin infections, and conjunctivitis.

Nettle

Nettle is also known by its Latin or homoeopathic name of *Urtica dioica* and comes from the *Urticacea* family. The leaf is used and should be collected when the plant is in flower.

The leaves are astringent, diuretic, and tonic. Nettle has the ability to increase the excretion of uric acid from the body. Uric acid is the compound that is produced from the breakdown of the DNA and RNA in the nucleus of cells. The main source of uric acid in your own body is the flesh foods and seeds that you eat, and in the form of sodium urate monohydrate, it is the substance of the needle-like crystals that form in joints such as those of the big toe, causing gout. Getting uric acid out of the body is obviously a good thing.

In spite of, or as homoeopaths would see it, because of, its ability to cause skin rashes, it is used in the treatment of eczema, dermatitis, and similar rashes, where it works well in combination with figwort and burdock.

As a side benefit, it has been used in the treatment of easy bleeding in general, and nosebleeds in particular. It is also helpful in the treatment of anemia that can result from such bleeding, as well as from other causes.

In spite of the prickles, you can eat nettle leaves as a vegetable or make them into a soup. There is no danger of a reaction once they have had boiling water poured on them or they have been cooked, but you would be wise to use rubber gloves while cleaning and preparing them for the pot.

- For an infusion, use one to three teaspoons of the chopped fresh leaves per cup. If you prefer the tincture, take ¼ to 1 teaspoon three times a day.

NETTLE SOUP

When picking the nettles, remember that they sting, and wear thick gloves. They are safe after they have been cooked. Pick 1⅓ cups of young nettles, remove the leaves from their stem, and wash. Like spinach leaves, they can then be cooked gently, relying on the remaining water left on their leaves, until they are soft.

Sauté 1 red onion, finely chopped, in olive oil. Clean and grate one potato, add to the onion, and sauté briefly. Add the washed nettle leaves and a generous bunch of fennel leaves, chopped. Finally, add 4 cups of stock, more or less depending on your preference, simmer for 15 minutes or until everything is well cooked, season, and serve.

Poke Root

Poke root, or *Phytolacca americana* from the *Phytolaccaceae* family, was discussed when we talked about herbs for the lymphatic system (p.160), but should be mentioned here as well, for it is an excellent blood cleanser and can also be used if toxins show up in the form of skin problems.

Red Clover

Trifolium pratense, one of the *Papilionaceae*, is an excellent herb for any Detox Regime. The flowers are easy to spot in any meadow and can be collected throughout their flowering season. If you are going to dry them, then collect them in full summer. They are an alterative, antispasmodic, and an expectorant.

First and foremost, red clover is a blood cleanser, exactly what we want for a general detoxing herb. As such, it is useful in the treatment of a range of skin problems, from the occasional pimple through full-blown acne, to cases of boils and other suppurating conditions. Use it with yellow dock for this purpose.

Second, it is an excellent expectorant and combines well with many other lung herbs to help expel mucus and to act as an appropriate alterative in congestion of the lungs and associated problems.

- The infusion is delicate and delicious. Allow one to three teaspoons of the dried flower per cup, more if using the fresh flowers, but clean them out first, as there may be insects inside. If you prefer the tincture, take ½ to 1 teaspoon three times a day.

BLOOD CLEANSING SALAD

Collect the leaves of blackberry, catnip, coriander, dandelion, greater celandine, nasturtium, pansy, primrose, and yellow dock. Clean and wash these, and add to the leaves of a head of lettuce. Add pumpkin seeds, some finely grated ginger, and toss with the Cleansing Salad Dressing. Place in a wooden bowl and decorate with the (edible) flowers of marigold, nasturtium, borage, chives, and red clover.

CLEANSING SALAD DRESSING

Combine three parts walnut oil with one part apple cider vinegar. Then add at least some of the following herbs: caraway and celery seeds; and the leaves of dill, fennel, mint, and thyme. The amounts and the ones selected will depend upon your own individual taste, but do be sure to include at least some crushed garlic.

Sarsaparilla

The root and rhizome of sarsparilla, which also goes by the happy name of *Smilax officinalis* and is from the *Liliacea* family, can be dug up and used at any time of the year. It is an alterative, antirheumatic, diuretic, and diaphoretic.

It is useful in the treatment of psoriasis, especially when it is the irritating form, and of eczema, and can be used in combination with burdock, cleavers, and yellow dock. It is particularly useful if these skin ailments are related to or the result of liver problems or poor liver function. Like nettle, it is useful in the treatment of gout, and it has helped in the treatment of leukorrhea.

- You need to make a decoction of this herb, allowing one to two teaspoons per cup and simmering for 10 minutes. Drink a cupful three times a day, or take ¼ to ½ teaspoon of the tincture three times a day.

Sassafras

The root bark of *Sassafras albidum* from the *Lauraceae* family is an alterative, carminative, diaphoretic, and diuretic. Its main use is in the treatment of skin problems such as eczema and psoriasis and it is generally used in combination with nettles and yellow dock. It can be used externally in the treatment and removal of head lice and other external parasites, and makes a good mouthwash and dentifrice.

- For the infusion, allow 1 to teaspoons of the herb per cup, or take ¼ to ½ teaspoon of the tincture three times a day.

Thuja

Thuja was discussed in the section on your lungs (p.181). So all we need do here is mention again that it is useful in the treatment of psoriasis, warts, and ringworm. It is particularly important to mention the latter two roles, as they are not dealt with by many of the other skin herbs we have mentioned. Apply it externally as a wash, a poultice, a cream or ointment.

Yellow Dock

Yellow dock, or *Rumex crispus* of the *Polygonaceae* family, offers another useful root for encouraging elimination and detoxification when problems show up with the skin. As we saw in the section on the liver (p.137), the root should be dug up in late summer or early autumn, and acts as an alterative, antiviral, cholagogue, and laxative.

It is particularly useful in situations involving acne or psoriasis, in association with problems of the liver or colon such as constipation, and we have already discussed it in this regard. For skin problems, it combines well with burdock and poke root; for constipation and associated liver problems, use it in combination with dandelion.

BLOOD-CLEANSING TEA FROM THE GARDEN

Collect equal parts of all or any of the following herbs. Most of them should be readily available if you have a garden or easy access to the countryside. Dandelion leaves, nettle leaves, primrose flowers and leaves, young elder shoots, red clover flowers, and peppermint. The latter is added mainly for flavor, and to clear your head. Chop the herbs, put in an attractive teapot, pour on boiling water, and allow to steep for a few minutes. If some of the leaves are too bitter for your taste, sweeten with a small amount of honey.

Antimicrobials

The next group of herbs helps to deal with unwanted micro-organisms on your skin. Inevitably there are millions of organisms all over your body. Every time you rub one hand on the other, you crush or brush off thousands, if not millions of them. Before you say that this makes your skin creep, it is worth noting that many of them are either beneficial or harmless. However, it is also true that there are some that can cause harm, particularly if you cut, burn or damage your skin in some way, and they can gain entry into your body. Even if they don't gain entry, they can cause localized skin problems such as acne pimples or sepsis.

Echinacea

Echinacaea has been considered in the section on the immune system (p.141). Because of this total cleansing effect, it is also useful in the treatment of skin problems. In particular, it is useful as a result of its action on bacterial or viral infections. Use it internally in the treatment of boils, or apply it as a poultice. It can also be used as a wash on any area of infection. Use it as a mouthwash, or spray onto gum infections.

Eucalyptus

Eucalyptus was mentioned briefly under the immune system (p.143). There are over three hundred types of eucalyptus, all indigenous to Australia, although in recent years some of them have been grown in other countries. A medicinal oil is extracted from the leaves that contains up to 85 percent eucalyptol from which a crystallizable resin can be extracted.

Eucalyptol is a very powerful antibacterial and antiseptic, it is also an aromatic, cardiac stimulant, decongestant, and diaphoretic.

For any form of skin infection, apply a diluted solution, either as a wash or as a damp pad under a dressing. It can be applied to ulcers, abrasions, cuts, and other wounds as an antiseptic.

Thuja

Thuja was discussed earlier (p.181) but also merits a mention here. Remember that it is useful in the treatment of such skin conditions as warts, psoriasis, and ringworm. It can also be useful in the treatment of fungal problems on the skin, such as athlete's foot, and problems with fungal infections of the nails.

Thyme

We considered thyme in the section on the digestive system (p.89). It is worth mentioning here that an infusion is helpful as an antiseptic on the skin if it is cut or infected. This is particularly useful to know, as there are few kitchens that don't have some of this herb.

Vulneraries, the Healing Herbs

We are still considering the skin here. However, it is wise to remember that the mucous membranes lining the internal cavities such as those of the digestive system, the respiratory system, and the genito-urinary system are in many (though certainly not all) ways similar to the skin on the outer parts of your body. Many herbs that help to heal the skin, after such toxic eliminations as boils, abscesses and pimples as well as after cuts and burns, are also effective in soothing and healing problems related to damaged mucous membranes.

Aloe Vera

Aloe vera, from the *Liliaceae* family, is such a useful plant that it is difficult to know in which section to put it. It is an anti-inflammatory, antimicrobial, immuno stimulant; and is anthelmintic, emmenagogue, vulnerary, and vermifuge. Externally it is a demulcent and vulnerary.

The leaf is used, but even this can be separated, and the parts used in different ways. The aloe leaf is a long, thin, tapering triangular shape that is generally a foot or more in length, several inches in width at the base, and up to an inch thick.

On the outside there is the epidermis or rind. This produces a bitter yellow juice that contains cathartics and purgatives and gave rise to the traditional use of aloes in herbal medicine, where it is quoted as being a laxative and cathartic. But this is only true when the whole leaf including this rind is used.

Second, there is the mucilaginous gel, which turns to a liquid juice on being exposed to the air. It is 98.5–99.5 percent water. While every attempt is usually made to extract only the pure gel, in practice a small amount of the juice from the rind may leak in during the extraction process, making some aloe vera juice laxative as well as healing. Any concentrating of the juice must be done without heat.

Third, there is the gel. It has properties similar to the juice but is used externally and can be applied directly to the skin.

Aloe vera is an antihistamine, so it can help with any allergic rashes. It is also a vasodilator and increases capillary permeability and the beneficial flow of blood to wounds. It helps to reduce the inflammation associated with many skin problems. It is an analgesic producing salicylates like those found in aspirin, so it can help to reduce the pain of cuts, burns, and abrasions. It inhibits some of the compounds that would otherwise lead to the formation of blood clots and reduce the movement of the beneficial white blood cells. The free movement of these white blood cells is important in dealing with local toxins. Furthermore, aloe vera is a general immune stimulant, helping the entire system to deal with infections.

It is a mild antimicrobial and vermifuge, not as strong, for instance, as garlic or golden seal, but it provides the additional benefits of markedly aiding the healing process. In this latter regard, it simulates the normal cellular growth and tissue reproduction and helps to restore the normal tissue structure. It can greatly reduce the risk of scar tissue formation and helps cuts and other wounds to heal normally.

Aloe vera has been used to help the healing of all sorts of skin problems. The gel can be applied to wounds, cuts, grazes, burns, and sunburn. If the problem is too serious to apply the gel, then aloe vera liquid can be sprayed on. This is particularly useful in the treatment of bad sunburn or serious burns.

Just as with so many herbs that are beneficial when applied to the skin, aloe vera is also beneficial for the mucous membranes. It is an excellent herb for the treatment of erosions of the digestive tract from top to bottom. This includes hiatus hernia, mild gastritis, stomach and duodenal ulcers, leaky gut, the problems caused by *Candida albicans* and other parasites, diverticulitis, colitis, and other inflammatory conditions of the small and large bowels. It can be applied externally to anal fissures and hemorrhoids to help the healing process.

For internal digestive problems, two to four tablespoons of the pure juice should be drunk three times a day. However, for acute problems and severe pain, it is often better to sip the tiniest amount of the liquid and to repeat this every minute or two so that there is an ongoing trickle of the juice down the digestive tract past the area concerned. This is particularly effective when the problem is in the esophagus and the stomach. After even a relatively short time, this will reduce the pain, particularly if it is taken in combination with slippery elm powder.

Aloe vera is an excellent healer in the genitourinary tract in the treatment of cystitis, vaginitis, thrush, or general abrasion. It combines well with propolis tincture for fungal problems or cystitis, and with marsh mallow as a demulcent.

Keep in mind that if the preparation you select contains the skin as well as the juice, it can be laxative and even a strong purgative. If used as the dried and concentrated herb for constipation, then monitor the dose carefully, as an excess can cause pain and cramping. If this happens, then use it in combination with a more gentle carminative.

Chickweed

Chickweed, or *Stellaria media* (in the *Caryophyllaceae* family), is well known to most gardeners as one of the common weeds they are forever trying to eradicate. This is a shame, as it is an excellent herb. The leaves and flowers can be collected at any time and are antirheumatic, vulnerary, and emollient.

Their main use is for skin problems, although chickweed is also useful in treatments for rheumatism. It is used both internally and externally in the treatment of eczema or dermatitis. Externally it is used as a wash, a poultice, a cream or ointment on itchy rashes, cuts, burns, and wounds of any sort. For this, it combines well with marsh mallow and golden seal.

- The infusion is made allowing two teaspoons per cup, and should be drunk three times a day.

Comfrey

Comfrey is another excellent herb when you want to promote the healing of skin problems. It can be used externally on the skin as a lotion, cream, or ointment. The leaves can also be used to make a poultice, which can be applied to clean wounds of all types, from small cuts to open ulcers and bedsores. A word of warning, however: do not use it on wounds that have not been cleaned, as the tissues may heal more rapidly than expected and so cover the dirt that is present, thus preventing proper cleansing and leading to possible sepsis. Similarly, do not use it over wounds that have been stitched with nondissolving stitches until the stitches themselves have been removed, or the healing may take place so rapidly it will become difficult to remove the stitches.

Golden Seal

We have already mentioned golden seal in a couple of sections (pp.93, 110, 159 and 186) so only brief mention will be made here of its beneficial effects on the skin. It is an excellent herb for a number of skin conditions including eczema, pruritis, and ringworm. It is important to realize that conditions such as eczema can have many causes including allergies and stress and nutrient deficiencies, and these problems should be attended to. Do not rely solely on an herbal ointment for the treatment. However, when all other activities are in place, then golden seal, taken internally and applied externally as an ointment, can greatly improve the rate of healing. The infusion can also be used externally as a wash for cuts, abrasions, and skin infections and in the treatment of conjunctivitis.

Horsetail

The stems of horsetail, or *Equisetam arvense,* should be cut in early summer and hung upside-down to dry. They are an excellent source of silica, an important nutrient for healthy skin. The

herb is an astringent, diuretic, and vulnerary. As such, it helps
to stem bleeding and to promote the healing of all types of cuts,
abrasions, and similar wounds. Horsetail can also be used as a
footbath for chilblains, or as a general bath in the treatment of
rheumatism.

- Make an infusion allowing two teaspoons per cup and leaving
  the mixture to infuse for 15 minutes. The tincture dose is ½
  to 1 teaspoon taken three times a day.

Irish Moss

All the names of this herb are evocative: Irish moss, *Chondrus
crispus,* or the dietary term, carragheen. Strictly speaking, it is
not an herb, but a seaweed, and it can be collected at low tide
from all the rocky coasts of northwest Europe and particularly, as
its name implies, from the coasts of Ireland.

The majority of the herb that is collected is used in the food
industry to make jellies and aspics and to give greater smooth-
ness to a number of food preparations. It is this capacity, as a
demulcent, that gives it its benefit in digestive problems such as
ulcers. It is used in the cosmetics industry and provides a soothing
demulcent quality to creams and lotions.

It also acts as an expectorant.

Linseed

We have discussed linseed under the digestive tract (p.104) and
the lungs (p.179). It is also useful for any skin problems you may
have. For one thing, by preventing constipation, it helps to prevent
the buildup of internal toxins that could then show up as skin
problems. It can also be used as an external poultice on such problems as boils, psoriasis, and shingles.

Marigold

Marigold is almost as well known by its Latin name of *Calendula
officinalis.* It's another of the many plants in the *Compositae* family
to have a health benefit and, as before, it is the petals that are

used. These should be collected in summer and dried with care to avoid bruising. Marigold is anti-inflammatory, astringent, vulnerary, antifungal, cholagogue, and emmenagogue.

It can be used on the skin both externally and internally. Externally it can be used as a poultice; or as a lotion, cream, or ointment for local trauma or damage. Because it is astringent, it will help to reduce bleeding time; as an anti-inflammatory and anti-fungal, it will help to reduce the risk of infections and inflammation; and as a vulnerary, it will help to promote healing. It can be used on cuts, burns, skin ulcers, and other wounds. It can also be applied to areas that have been bruised and sprained, to reduce the trauma, inflammation, and swelling. The effect of the local application can be enhanced if the herb is also taken internally. For skin infections, it can be combined with cat's claw and golden seal.

It is kind to the mucous membranes as well as the skin, including those of the digestive system, another part of the Detox Regime. It is helpful when dealing with stomach and duodenal ulcers, inflammatory problems such as ileitis and colitis, and to help repair the damage to the intestinal lining caused by the mold *Candidia albicans*. It works well in combination with aloe vera juice, slippery elm powder, and marsh mallow.

Similarly, it will help the urinary system and is used in the treatment of cystitis, urethritis, and vaginitis; and also as an antifungal for vaginal thrush. For these purposes, it can be used as a douche.

- For an infusion, allow 1 to 2 teaspoons of the herb per cup, or take ½ to 1 teaspoon of the tincture three times a day.

Marsh Mallow Root

Both the root and the leaves of marsh mallow, or *Althea officinalis* (a Malvaceae), are used. The leaves should be collected in summer after the plant has flowered, and the roots in autumn. Both the root and the leaves are demulcent, diuretic, and emollient. In addition, the root is a vulnerary, and the leaves are expectorant.

Both parts of the plant can be used externally on the skin as an emollient, and in addition, the roots will help any skin lesions to heal. Use it in conditions where there are acne pimples, boils, abscesses, or ulcers. In practice, you will probably get marsh mallow cream or ointment that will contain both parts of the plant.

The herb is also useful, again as an emollient and vulnerary, in the digestive system for situations where there is inflammation. These may range from mouth ulcers through hiatus hernia, gastritis, and stomach and duodenal ulcers, to ileitis and colitis. It is best used in combination with slippery elm powder and aloe vera juice.

For the same reasons, it is useful in combination with coltsfoot and horehound, for coughs, catarrhal inflammations, and bronchitis in the respiratory system; and for urethritis and cystitis in the urinary tract.

- A decoction can be made from the root, allowing one teaspoon per cup, or make an infusion of leaves, again allowing one teaspoon per cup. If you prefer the tincture, take ¼ to 1 teaspoon three times a day.

Slippery Elm

As the name implies, the elm tree *Ulmus fulva* (an Ulmaceae) or *Ulmus campestris* is used (see p.105). It is an astringent and a gentle-acting demulcent and emollient.

It is also an excellent herb for soothing the digestive system. The mucilaginous substances are not broken down in the digestive processes, and they combine with the fluids in the digestive tract to make, in effect, an internal bandage, covering the mucous membranes with a protective layer. The mucilage then stimulates normal mucosal secretion, which further aids the healing process.

It can be used for any pain in the digestive system that involves damage to the mucous membrane. Such problems include esophagitis, hiatal hernia, gastritis, gastric and duodenal ulcers, Crohn's disease, intestinal thrush, ileitis, diverticulitis, and colitis, plus those related to constipation, diarrhea, and hemorrhoids. It will give even better results if combined with aloe vera juice. If you are using it for the treatment of constipation or diarrhea, it is best combined with a slightly more effective laxative such as powdered psyllium hulls.

For skin lesions, slippery elm powder can be made into a poultice and put on abscesses, boils, ulcers, pimples, and open sores.

Make a paste by mixing the powder with boiling water. Allow this to cool until it can just be placed on the skin.

- For problems in the digestive tract, take one to three teaspoons before meals. Most of my patients find that the best way to do this is to mash it into a banana. It can also be made into a nutritious drink by preparing a combination of one part slippery elm powder to 10 parts of water or milk. Mix this into a paste, bring to a boil, and simmer for 10 minutes. Flavor it with cinnamon, nutmeg, or mac;e and sweeten with honey if desired.

Witch Hazel

Witch hazel is frequently given its homoeopathic name of *Hamamelis virginiana (Hamameliadaceae)*. The bark is collected in spring, after sprouting, and the leaves are collected in the summer. It acts as an astringent.

Its main use is to stem or reduce bleeding, whether internally or external. Thus, it is used externally in the treatment of cuts and wounds and internally in the treatment of bruises, sprains with swelling, hemorrhoids, and varicose veins.

- You can make an infusion using one teaspoon of the herb per cup. The tincture dose is ¼ to ½ teaspoon three times a day.

+++ PART V +++

Developing Your Own Detox Regime

CHAPTER 15

The Four-Week Detox Regime

BEFORE YOU EVEN START ON A DETOX REGIME, you should consider just how much effort you are prepared to put into it. Obviously, the more changes you make, the more benefits you are likely to experience. Equally, making changes may seem to be simply a case of giving up things you like on the one hand, and having to do things that take time and trouble on the other. At some point, you will decide the effort is greater than the perceived benefit.

Try to establish just where that line comes for you. I have had hundreds of patients over the years who have said such things as, "I would love to lose weight," or "I would love to have more energy," or "I would love to be healthier," or "I would love to feel more alert and less lethargic." Of course they would love these things. They would love the end result; they would not necessarily love the process.

Very few people love losing weight. They would love to be slim, sure enough, but very few people enjoy the process of dieting, eating less, and progressively losing the weight. Many know that fat- and sugar-laden foods are not giving them the nutrients they need for energy. They know that a quick takeaway or snack is not going to give them the energy they need, but they often feel that making a proper meal for themselves is just too much effort.

More patients than I can count find taking supplements a bother, and eventually say they haven't got the time or that they forgot. Yet it is these supplements to their poor diet that can help them achieve better health.

Similarly, few people want the bother, as they see it, of going on a Detox Regime, yet they want to feel lithe, physically healthy and clean, and mentally alert.

It is terribly boring to hear "no pain, no gain," but it is certainly true that what you have been doing in your life up till now, the food you've been eating, the fluids you've been drinking (or not drinking), the chemicals you've allowed into your home and your body, and various other lifestyle habits have brought you to where you are. It is reasonably certain that, since you are reading this, you are not altogether happy with where that is. So some changes are in order. As I used to say to seminar students:

If you don't change the direction in which you are headed, you will land up where you are going.

Patients often say to me: "If I eat a good diet most days, surely it won't matter if I binge on junk food on Sundays." Or, "I mostly eat well, surely the occasional dessert won't matter." To which my reply usually goes something like this: "You work, you get paid at the end of each week or each month. How would you feel if your boss said to you from time to time, 'Look, most weeks your pay packet is full, but this week some of the bank notes have been replaced with bits of junk mail. I hope you won't mind. After all, I usually pay you most of what we agreed.' Would you mind? Of course you would. So does your body. It may not make its response obvious immediately, but in time it will gradually work less and less well for you until it stops and forces you to pay it attention. This is usually in a way that causes you significant harm and distress. The damage may or may not be reparable. It is much easier to prevent than to cure."

It is now time for you to consider just where you stand on this. There is little point in setting yourself up for failure by setting goals that require input from you that you are unwilling to make. At the end of the day, you will simply not have achieved those goals, and you will have failure to berate yourself with. On the other hand, if you don't make a concerted effort, you will not make the improvements in your health for which you are looking.

Detoxing is not a random, one-day affair. You should set aside *four weeks* to put the following program into action. Then plan to follow a maintenance program, or a new lifestyle regime, so that you do not need to go through the process all over again some months or years later.

Be realistic, then push just that tiny bit further. Envision what it will take, what you are prepared to do, and the results you can hope for. Then get started.

There are several parts to your Detox Regime. Inevitably, you must tailor it to your own individual needs.

Three things are required of you:

- reduce your intake of toxins
- improve the quality of your diet
- use the herbs or any other supplements that are specific to your own particular needs

There is little point in taking a lot of cleansing herbs while you are still pouring the toxins into your system.

Herbs can play an invaluable role in the Detox Regime, either to prevent harm or to treat problems. However, they cannot do it all on their own. Correcting your diet is a powerful step to feeling cleaner and healthier; so is changing your lifestyle.

If you have no specific symptoms or problems but just feel generally somewhat sluggish and as if you need a good cleanout, then choose one or two of the major herbs from each section of the Top Ten Tinctures in the next chapter. Keep in mind, however, that almost inevitably, there are several different herbs that can accomplish your purpose, and the final selection can be up to you. It may even be dictated by availability or other practical considerations.

If you have a specific reason for wanting a Detox Regime, then your selection of herbs will be slanted in that direction. If, for instance, you are generally in good health but have problems with your digestive system, with your skin, or have respiratory problems, then you will want to focus on herbs that improve that particular system. However, I would suggest that you do also pay attention to the rest of your body, as it could well be, for instance, a minor degree of immune incompetence that is a contributing factor in your skin problems.

Reduce Your Intake of Toxins

We discussed toxins in Part II. As I've said, there is little point in cleaning your system out while at the same time loading in the toxins. So this is the time to clean up your act. Take a look at what you are doing, the chemicals to which you are exposing yourself, and the additives and chemicals you are consuming. Reduce them to a minimum.

It is worth reminding yourself, from time to time, of the need to do this. It is all too easy, in our society, to slip back into your old ways, to say to yourself that other people do so and so, so it can't matter, or that "just once" this or that doesn't matter. But it does. Each fat-laden snack that replaces a balanced meal of fruits and vegetables gives your body something more to cope with. Each time you buy organic food rather than chemically treated food, it saves your body having to cope with the accompanying toxins.

The same is true of each time you go into polluted environments, spray chemicals around your house, use your mobile phone, or sit close to and directly in front of the television.

Every small step you take to cleaning up your act will improve your health and well-being. Each tiny intake of toxins is one more load on the system.

Make a plan. I am strongly in favor of writing your thoughts down. List the things you are willing to do. Then at the end of each week or month, you can review this list and see if you are doing what you promised.

Ask yourself what you are prepared to do. You may not be prepared to stay out of smoky pubs or stop using your mobile phone. But you may be willing to angle the television slightly sideways, buy yourself a water purifier, throw out all those spray cans of household cleaner and insect killers, and buy organic cleaning materials. Look around your home, your workplace, and the places where you socialize. Make your decisions, write them down, and then act on them. Most important, maintain these activities.

The more toxins you remove from your environment, the fewer you have to deal with inside your own body.

Improve the Quality of Your Diet

Herbs have a great deal to offer, but they will have to work overtime if you don't improve your diet. Again, some soul-searching and some decision-making is required. Remember, if you don't make the changes; you won't improve your health, but if you make rash promises to yourself and then don't keep them, you will only create a sense of guilt or failure. I can only tell you the absolutes, what you absolutely should do for maximum health.

I can't make the compromise decisions for you, as only you can do that.

Ideally, all your food should be organically produced. You may decide to make sure this is the case, or you may decide you can't afford it. To which I can honestly reply, if you think staying healthy is expensive, think about the cost of being ill. Buying organic might raise the price of your shopping basket up by a few dollars, but what do you currently spend that extra money on that you could do without? Perhaps it's that extra makeup when you already have a drawer full, that extra outfit that you'll wear just once, a couple of drinks that you really didn't need and that have left you with a hangover, or a purchase from the candy store or pastry shop.

If you don't buy organic food, then at least concentrate on what I call "individual" foods. These are single foods that are recognizable as some part of a plant or animal. Buy fresh tomatoes, onions, garlic, and herbs, for instance, and make your own tomato sauce instead of buying a processed, red-colored sauce with additives. Remember, each time two or more foods are put together in a packet, tin, jar, tube, or bottle, there is the chance for the manufacturer to add one or more chemicals to it to improve the color, consistency, flavor, or shelf life, while at the same time giving you one or more toxins to deal with and thus probably damaging your health. You may say you don't have time to do this. I suggest you don't have time *not* to.

I once worked it out with a patient. If she allowed herself 20 minutes each morning to eat a fresh fruit salad and yogurt for breakfast, and put together a lunch box of vegetables and some lean protein to take to work for lunch, and saved the 5 minutes she spent shopping for a croissant and cappuccino on the way to work and the 10 minutes it took to go out at lunchtime, buy a sandwich and return to work she would not only save herself money — which could go to the organic supermarket — she would also save time. The extra 5 minutes each working morning, 5 days a week, for 48 weeks in the year amounted to a total of 20 hours per year. She had already spent that much time off work sick, and now she had the traveling time coming to see me, the time in the consultation, and more time traveling home.

Even if you were to spend an extra 15 minutes a day looking

after your health, shopping for better food, and preparing better meals, and if you did this every single day for the next 30 years, that would only add up to a total of 2,730 hours, or 113.75 days, or 16.25 weeks, or approximately four months. You would almost certainly lengthen your life by that much if not more, probably a lot more, and you would feel better and spend less time seeing doctors or naturopaths in the bargain. You would also have saved yourself a small fortune in over-the-counter medications, in cold remedies, headache-blocking painkillers, and digestive aids.

So be wary of saying you don't have time or money to take better care of your health or shop for and cook better food for yourself. You don't have time not to, even if that time is some-time in the future.

Perhaps you like to eat out a lot, in restaurants or with friends, and blame that on your poor diet. Yet eating well in restaurants can be surprisingly easy. All right, so you probably won't find organic food, except in a few specialized restaurants, but you can make wise choices. It is just as easy to order a salad for a starter as a puff pastry with a small amount of smoked salmon in it and a sauce over it. Or order one of my favorites — a plate of spinach or some other vegetable. For the main course, it is as easy to order a simple grilled fish or meat with several vegetables as it is to order a chicken-pot pie or even fish or meat lathered in a rich creamy sauce. Who needs fries? And remember what was said about the toxins in those fats. Have a salad instead. If you must have a dessert, have fresh fruit. If that is not available, then decline; you've probably had plenty to eat anyway.

What about friends? Do they invite you over and offer nothing but buns and pizzas, or trays laden with chips and sweets? I simply tell all my friends that I don't have a sweet tooth. I have avoided all the sugar-laden desserts at dinner parties by this strategy, and they now tend to make a habit of offering some fresh fruit as part of the meal, better for me but better for all of them, too.

Decide what changes you are willing to make. The chances are that you already know what you should be doing. Now is the time to put those ideas, along with whatever you learn here, into prac-tice. If you are serious about improving your diet and not sure quite what to do, this could be a good time to get advice, either from a professional or by consulting some of the many available good books on what constitutes a healthy diet.

When you decide just how many improvements you are going to make to your diet, there are two things to consider: your starting diet and your maintenance diet.

At the start of a Detox Regime, you probably want to get quick results. You will be looking for reassurance that all you are doing is producing a result, and that the effort is worth it. It may also be that your starting problem is sufficiently noticeable, painful, or uncomfortable that it warrants a significant change in what you are doing. For this reason, I suggest that for the first week you go on a fairly restricted cleansing diet. You will find out shortly just what this means — although you may find it is actually less restrictive than you had feared. Then over the four weeks of the Detox Regime, the diet gets progressively more and more liberal, more and more back to a general diet on which you can probably base your future diet.

After that, you will find suggestions for a maintenance diet. This will be the time for you to decide just how healthy or casual that diet will be.

Your Own Choice of Herbs

As there will be no direct conversation between you and me, I cannot design your specific choice of herbs. However, I have already given you more than sufficient information to allow you to make your own choices. In the next chapter, I will outline a group of herbs that make up a good, overall cleansing and Detox Regime. I will also give you some pointers as to how to construct your own selection of herbs.

This is another time to be honest with yourself. There is little point in going out and buying 20 different tinctures if, after a week or two, you are going to lose interest in the whole process. If you are serious about a Detox Regime, then go ahead and decide which tinctures you need and purchase them.

If you are uncertain, or feel insecure working with tinctures, then visit your local health-food store, or write to a mail-order herbal supplier and see what they have available as prepared combinations of herbs, possibly in capsule or tablet form, to deal with your specific problem. Having read this far, you are in a position to make an informed choice as to which of the several combinations they probably have to offer that will be best suited to your needs. You might find, for instance, that you can buy capsules of herbs for your lungs that include horehound and lobelia; and another remedy that includes coltsfoot and peppermint. If you have a deep bronchial cough that seems to come from the depths of your chest with a tendency toward asthma, you would now know to choose the one with horehound and lobelia. If, on the other hand, you had a ticklish cough with lots of wet phlegm and blocked sinuses, you might choose the one with coltsfoot and peppermint.

If you are still more unsure about your commitment to a full Herbal Detox Regime, then you could start by building your program around the herbs that are available in the culinary sections (Chapter 18 — Detox from the Kitchen), cooking herbs that you can continue to use for flavor, and herbal teas that you can continue to enjoy for their inherent refreshment, if nothing else.

There are more ways than one to go about a Detox Regime. The trick is to find out what suits you. Remember, though, that the more effort you put into it and the more positive changes you make, the more you are likely to get out of it. The fewer toxins you take in, the better your diet, and the more thoughtful your herbal regime, the healthier you are likely to be.

In the instructions and guidelines given here, you may feel that I am being too strict. A number of my patients certainly say that this is the case. However, I see it as my job to inform you of what you can do to achieve the best possible results, rather than to condone the errors that contribute to ill health and try to assure you that you will still be all right.

Getting Ready

If you like to ease gently into things, this is the time to do it. If you hate waste and want to eat up what is in your refrigerator and cupboards, so be it. You may say this is the food you have been eating for years, surely one week more or less won't make all that much difference. To an extent, this is true; but make sure you don't lose the impetus to make the changes, and don't use this as an excuse to delay the start of your Detox Regime and keep following your old ways.

If you really want to clear out your cupboards in a hurry, have a party. You could argue that, since you now recognize that these foods are harmful, that will be harming your friends. Don't worry. These are probably the foods that they all eat anyway, and will continue to eat. And you could always take the opportunity to tell them just why you are having the party and what you are planning to do — they might even join you.

You may feel that you need time to shop for the new foods you are going to be eating and for the herbs you need. Certainly this can be the case. However, try to make a start, concentrate on increasing your intake of fruit and vegetables and cutting down on processed foods, fats and sugars, giving your body a taste of what is to come.

A Word about Water

You are going to be advised to drink water, lots of it. If you have dipped in to this book at this point, it is worth repeating that unfortunately your normal tap water is no longer good enough — it contains too many chemicals from chlorine to aluminium, and too many other toxins, in spite of all the so-called purification it undergoes.

You could, of course, buy bottled water. If you do, you should use this not only for drinking, but for making herb teas and infusions and for cooking with. You don't want the water your brown rice absorbs to be full of the same toxins you are trying to eliminate from your body. All this water, at ½ to ¾ gallon a day minimum, can be quite expensive. So this could be a good time to buy a water purifier.

A water filter would be a help, although filters have many drawbacks. For one thing, they only remove some of the toxins, and as they absorb toxins, they become more and more clogged up, and can thus eventually become a source of toxins themselves. For the best results, I recommend a reverse osmosis system. These are somewhat more expensive in initial outlay than filters, but give better results and are usually less expensive to maintain.

Another Word about Chewing

Proper digestion is important if you want to have a healthy digestive tract, and you will recall that everything else stems from that. For proper digestion, it is important that you get a good flow of digestive juices. This happens when you work up the saliva in your mouth, eat slowly, and chew your food thoroughly. Not only does this get the breakdown of food off to a good start, leaving less work for your stomach and intestines, it also gives the rest of your digestive tract time to get into action. It gives your stomach time to produce the required amount of acid, your pancreas to produce sufficient digestive enzymes and alkali fluids, and your gallbladder to release sufficient bile. All this in turn stimulates the peristaltic action that will propel your food through the system at the correct rate.

When you feel ready, no matter what day it is, get started.

Week One

This week is particularly important if you feel you are very toxic; if you have been used to a high consumption of processed foods, fats, alcohol, tea, coffee, and chocolate; if you smoke cigarettes; and so forth. It is the start of the serious detox part of your Detox Regime.

There is no need to hibernate, but if you can take things easy this week, it is helpful. This is not the week to be doing a heavy round of social entertaining, going away on business trips, or burning the midnight oil to meet a deadline.

This is the week to listen to your appetite and eat only when hungry. Do have snacks if you seriously need them, but have no more than two courses at any one meal. Don't overeat. You will find that the foods allowed this week are surprisingly filling and satisfying, although they are generally low in calories. You will also find, since the suggested foods are relatively high-fiber, bulky foods as well as being low in calories, that you start to lose weight.

The weight loss may be hastened by the loss of unwanted fluid that you have been retaining. As you increase your intake of fruits and vegetables and cut down on your intake of salty foods, you will find that your sodium and potassium balance changes, your fluid balance changes, and you lose the excess fluid you have been storing. This could amount to two pounds or more. Don't get too excited, though. You can only lose this once as you normalize the state of your tissues. From then on, any weight loss comes about from eating less and eating better.

Since this is the beginning of your Detox Regime, this is the time when it is most important to get organically grown food if you possibly can. This is the week to make that effort. The longer the period of time you can stay on food without the added chemicals, the better.

If your fruits and vegetables are not organically grown, it is important that they are peeled and the peel discarded. There are several "natural" solutions you can buy to clean fruits and vegetables. They help to remove not only the dirt and bacteria, but some of the surface pesticides and other chemicals as well. This is the time to find and use them; in fact, this is something you should continue to do even after the four weeks of this Detox Regime.

During this week, your diet should consist of fresh fruit and vegetables, fresh herbs, spices, brown rice, fish, and a small amount of virgin olive oil. If you are allergic to rice, use buckwheat instead.

- the fruit and vegetables will alkalize your body and provide most of your trace nutrients,
- the fish will ensure you have sufficient protein and some essential fatty acids
- the brown rice will ensure you feel satisfied, and provide fiber and B-group vitamins
- the olive oil will give you the essential fatty acids and will stimulate your gallbladder.

You will also be including all the herbs you choose in the next chapter. Some of these you will add to your food; others you will drink as teas; and still others you may be taking as capsules, tablets, or tinctures.

Make frequent use of vegetables such as garlic, onion, artichoke, beets, and the cabbage family. These are good for your liver, which is going to be working hard to help you get rid of the stored toxins. The onions and garlic will discourage molds and other parasites in your digestive tract.

It is important that you have three good bowel motions a day. Very few people achieve this on the normal Western diet, with its high content of processed foods and low-fiber content. So for this Regime, it is important that you include some bulking agents in your diet to start stimulating your colon into activity. You may very well need these in addition to the extra fiber you will be eating as a result of your increased intake of vegetables.

Adding linseeds to your diet is an easy way to achieve this. They can be sprinkled over salads or incorporated into vegetable dishes. Add them to food at the last minute, just prior to serving. If the seeds are added to liquids ahead of time, they are likely to thicken up and spoil the texture of the dish. If you prefer psyllium hulls or slippery elm powder, you can, of course, use them instead.

Build your diet around the following outline.

Breakfast

Have fresh fruit or fresh fruit salad. If this does not satisfy you and you feel you must have something more, then have some cooked brown rice with it, or some brown rice cereal, such as puffed brown rice. Or, you could eat one or two rice cakes if those appeal to you.

Lunch

Have a fresh vegetable salad with some fish. Make a salad dressing from olive oil and either lemon juice or vinegar, and incorporate into that as many of your chosen herbs as are appropriate. Include fresh herbs in your salad such as dandelion leaves, nasturtium leaves and flowers, watercress, parsley, and seeds such as celery and dill. Include crushed or chopped fresh garlic. See the chapter on culinary herbs (p.236) to help you make your selection. Combine this with an awareness of the flavors you enjoy. It is important to make this Regime as pleasurable as possible, and you can do this by paying attention to the variety of flavors herbs have to offer as well as their healing benefits.

Fresh fish would be much better than canned fish, but if you must choose the latter, choose sardines or salmon rather than tuna, and make sure it is in plain water or olive oil and not some other sauce.

Dinner

Start off with a clear, homemade vegetable soup. You can use some meat or fish bones for this, add vegetables and a range of herbs. Make sure that you don't overcook the vegetables. Make the meat or fish stock first, if you want one, adding the herbs and spices from the start. Strain, and then add the vegetables and cook until they are just tender. Or, start your meal with a fresh vegetable salad consisting of lots of fresh green leaves and an herbal dressing.

Your main course should consist of a large plate of steamed fresh vegetables with fish, brown rice, and a side salad; yes, again, another salad. These salads are a serious part of your Detox Regime. Since you probably enjoy eating, you might as well prolong the experience by eating lots of fresh salads.

Or, you might want to do a stir-fry with the vegetables, and remember to include all the herbs with them. If you are doing a stir-fry, you may want to add slices of fresh ginger; or you could make a curry and add a variety of spices, including cayenne, coriander, cardamom, and a generous amount of turmeric, which helps your digestion and provides other benefits. If your garden provides them, add fresh nettles. Make a pesto-like sauce from a cupful of finely chopped herbs, some crushed garlic, and olive oil. Serve this with the brown rice to add flavor. You will find you can incorporate a wide range of herbs this way.

If you want a dessert, make one from fresh fruit and herbs. Try adding peppermint leaves to a fresh fruit salad, or cinnamon or nutmeg to apples or pears.

Snacks

Have some fresh fruit or raw vegetable pieces. You can dress the latter up as crudités with a dip made from olive oil and fresh lemon juice. Use this as another chance to build in some of your herbs. Or nibble on a dish of seeds that will give you some of the benefits you are after. These could be the carminative seeds such as cardamom or cumin or, if candida is a problem, it could include pumpkin seeds.

Beverage

Drink aloe vera juice once or twice each day. Drink a daily total of at least ½ gallon of water or similar fluids. This can include water, fruit juices, herbal teas, dandelion coffee and soups. It does not include any alcohol, soft drinks, tea, or regular coffee.

This is your first week's diet. It may seem very restrictive, however it is not unhealthy, far from it. It is about as close to our ancestral Stone Age diet as we can get, and this proved to be a healthy diet for humans for many, many thousands of years. You could certainly stay on this regime for the rest of your life and feel all the better for it. It is probable that few people will choose to do that, but if you are feeling and enjoying the benefits of it, you can certainly stay on it for as long as you like.

Week Two

The emphasis this week should still be on fresh fruits, salads, and lots of vegetables. However, unless you choose to stay on last week's diet, you can now add other foods if you wish. You can include legumes such as red kidney beans and lentils, and soy bean products such as soy milk and soy yogurt. You can add eggs and chicken to your choice of proteins. Add other grains such as millet, quinoa, or spelt; but not wheat, barley, oats, rye, or corn. You can include raw nuts and seeds in addition to pumpkin seeds. Keep in mind that these should all be raw, not roasted or coated in fats that have been overheated. Eat "Tasty Nibbles" instead (see next page).

Structure your meals in the same general way as in Week One. Be sure to drink as much water and to take the herbs you have chosen.

TASTY NIBBLES

Heat olive oil in a pan gently; you do not want it to smoke. Add cayenne pepper, powdered coriander, cumin, fenugreek, mace, dill, and crushed garlic (avoid paprika and turmeric as they can stain your fingers and your clothes); add celery powder or celery salt, freshly ground black pepper, and any other spices you desire. Heat gently for five minutes. Then add your favorite nuts or seeds.

For this week of your Detox Regime, you should use pumpkin seeds, cucumber seeds, sunflower seeds, and linseeds. Later you can add the nuts — but not peanuts, never peanuts. Peanuts are not, strictly speaking, a nut; they are a bean. They contain an antinutritive factor that blocks your own digestion and makes them, and other foods you eat at the same time, difficult to digest. In addition, they commonly contain a toxic and carcinogenic mold called aphlotoxin.

Week Three

Yet again, the emphasis should still be on fresh fruits, salads, and lots of vegetables. And again, you can remain on the diet of either Week One or Week Two for as long as you like. However, if you wish to expand your food selection, you can now incorporate all the other grains, with the exception of wheat. You can include oats and oat cakes, for instance, and have rye breads. You can also incorporate meat, but avoid sausages and other processed meats. Continue to avoid dairy products. Both dairy products and wheat can produce unwanted mucus in susceptible people, and this is something you want to avoid on a Detox Regime.

Again, structure your meals in the same general way as in Week One. Be sure to drink as much water and to continue taking the herbs you have chosen.

Week Four and the Future

You've done the work. It is now time to establish a lifestyle that will suit you in the future. You do not want to unravel what you have achieved. Keep focusing on fresh fruits, vegetables, and salads. You can now bring wheat and dairy products back into your diet, if you wish, although it is probably wise to limit the amounts, particularly of the hard cheeses. You should still leave out highly processed foods, foods laden with sugar or saturated fats, foods based on refined white flour, and white-flour products.

Continue to incorporate beneficial herbs and spices in your diet — make them a permanent part of your lifestyle — drink plenty of water, and replace tea and coffee with herb teas or dandelion coffee on a permanent basis.

If you want to drink alcohol, drink wine rather than spirits. Remember to have a wine glass full of mineral water beside your wine glass and drink that, rather than the wine, most of the time.

✦✦✦ ✦✦✦

+ CHAPTER 16 +

Your Top Ten Tinctures

YOU KNOW WHAT TO EAT. It is now time to choose the herbs to use for this Detox Regime. In this chapter, I have chosen a selection of herbs for you. For this purpose, I am assuming that you have no specific symptoms but simply want to undertake a general Detox Regime. I have thus chosen what I consider to be some of the best herbs, one for each part of your body or each body system. The list is not set in concrete. If you prefer milk thistle to dandelion, or echinacea to cat's claw, you can make the appropriate changes.

Do keep in mind that I am assuming you have no overt or particular symptoms and are in generally good health. You may be feeling a bit run down, a bit in need of some fine-tuning, and a general perk-up, but would not call yourself "ill." I am assuming that you want a bit of a spring clean and a chance to support your body so that it does not develop any health problems. If you have specific problems, then by using Part IV, you can adapt your choice of herb to your specific health needs.

Even when people feel generally well, there may be some minor problems or some developing problems. I have had dozens of patients who have come into the practice saying that there is nothing particularly wrong with them; they just don't feel quite right. This is a program that could benefit them.

Herb No. 1 (Gentian Root)

Include a sialogogue or bitters to ensure that your digestive system gets off to a good start. If you want culinary rather than medical herbs, you could choose from cayenne, ginger, or thyme, particularly if you like their flavor and they fit into your meal plan and can be used as part of your diet. Otherwise, you might want to choose gentian root, one of the most effective sialogogues.

Because it is also a bitter herb and gastric stimulant, it will activate your stomach as well; and because it is also a cholagogue, its benefit will flow down to your liver and gallbladder and hence, your whole intestinal system.

Make sure you include in your diet some of the many carminatives (see Herbal Functions table, p.57) from among the culinary herbs and spices to ensure you do not suffer from gas, and drink one or two cups of peppermint tea throughout the day to relieve any possibility of trapped wind.

Herb No. 2 (Milk Thistle)

Add an herb for your liver. Milk thistle and dandelion are the obvious candidates. I suggest you add dandelion to your diet in several different ways. It is an excellent herb for your liver and, as a significant cholagogue, improves peristalsis and helps to prevent constipation. Add the leaves to salads and vegetable dishes, and drink the root, ground up and roasted, as a coffee.

You might feel that since gentian root is also a cholagogue, dandelion is redundant. Not at all. The healthy and efficient functioning of your liver is such an important part of your Detox Regime that you need an herb that is a true hepatic and benefits your liver in many different ways. Remember that as well as stimulating your liver and gallbladder, dandelion is also a diuretic, laxative, and tonic — just what we want.

This leaves a place for milk thistle in the Top-Ten Tinctures, for your liver. It may seem that a lot of attention is being paid to your liver, but it needs it; it has a lot of work to do. As a cholagogue, demulcent, antioxidant, and galactogogue, milk thistle will support your liver, soothe any parts of your digestive tract that need healing, and provide invaluable antioxidant activity for further protection from toxins.

Herb No. 3 (Rhubarb Root)

By including plenty of vegetables, salads, and fruit in your diet, and by adding linseeds, you should be able to achieve the normal three soft bowel motions a day. The actions of gentian root and dandelion should further support this. Drinking rosehip tea as well as dandelion coffee and eating horseradish sauce — your own homemade variety, of course — will also help, as will turning some of your meals into curries with cayenne or chili.

However, at the start of your Detox Regime, you may need some extra help. The herb you choose will depend on just how constipated you are. If you need extra help, I would suggest rhubarb root, as it is not only laxative but it is also astringent and will deal with any possible bleeding and help to tone up the muscles of the walls of the colon, thus helping to normalize peristaltic action. On top of that, it is a bitter herb and will contribute to good digestion in the stomach.

Herb No. 4 (Cat's Claw)

You need something to stimulate and support your immune system. Although echinacea is popular, I have chosen *cat's claw* as a better herb to take as part of a long-term prophylactic program. It supports your immune system in the best possible way. As an adaptogen, it helps, via hormonal responses, to balance and adjust your immune response. It is anti-inflammatory, antiviral, and parasiticide, so it will help as a digestive antimicrobial as well as increasing your immune system's action on viruses and bacteria. As an anti-inflammatory, it will help to settle any inflammation in your digestive tract, as well as systemic inflammations. It is an antioxidant, a heart tonic, helps to balance female hormone disturbances, and is used in the treatment of arthritis. It is clearly too important an herb to exclude.

Be sure to add plenty of garlic and nasturtium leaves to your diet, and incorporate them both in cooking and in salads. Add generous amounts of thyme when the flavor is appropriate.

I am not including a febrifuge herb in this program as, by our starting definition, you have no significant symptoms and so no fever. If, during the course of the Detox Regime your temperature does increase, then there are several culinary diaphoretics you can include to maximize the loss of toxins via the skin in perspiration or sweat. These include cayenne and ginger, so think about eating curries, or drink either ginger or peppermint tea and add oregano to your salad herbs.

Herb No. 5 (Poke Root)

For your lymphatic system, it is hard to go past poke root; it is such a good herb for swollen glands all over your body and has so many other side benefits. It is anticatarrhal and will help to clear out the nose, sinuses, and lungs; and is a purgative, so it will add its support to treat constipation.

Herb No. 6 (Bucchu)

Your kidneys will be getting a boost from the dandelion leaves you are adding to your diet. To help them further, you could include either buchu or couch grass. I have selected the former, as couch grass is better used as an infusion rather than as a tincture. Bucchu is an antiseptic and diuretic and one of the best herbs for your kidneys. It will help to prevent infections of the kidneys and urinary tract and will encourage the loss of any waste fluids your body is holding, encouraging the flushing out of toxins.

There's no shortage of diuretics to add to your diet either. Make sure you add cucumber — the flesh and the seeds — and celery seeds, chervil, and fresh corn silk if you can get it, to your diet for their diuretic action. Horseradish and mustard will also contribute, as they too are diuretic. So will nettle leaves, but make sure you cook them — the raw leaves in a salad would leave a lasting impression on your mouth (I have known it to happen).

Herb No. 7 (Coltsfoot)

You want a good lung herb and expectorant to eliminate catarrh and clear toxins out from the lungs. Coltsfoot is a good choice. It is an excellent lung herb and combines well with other herbs. It is antitussive, anticatarrhal, and expectorant, and so it is helpful if you do have or develop a cough as part of your detoxing process. It is demulcent and so will help soothe damaged mucous membranes, and is also a diuretic and benefits your urinary tract. Although lobelia may be a more powerful lung herb, it is used best when there are specific lung problems, which we are currently assuming to be absent, and has fewer side benefits to other parts of the body than does coltsfoot.

Herb No. 8 (Red Clover)

Now we need an herb to help your skin. The choice here is difficult, as there are so many excellent herbs. If you have a garden, nettle and cleavers can be incorporated into your diet. In addition to cleansing your skin, burdock would benefit your digestive system and is a diuretic. Poke root would also benefit your lymphatic system, but it already has a place in the team, so I am choosing red clover because it is an excellent alterative, is a good expectorant to expel unwanted mucus that may be produced as you start to Detox, and because it combines well with a range of other herbs. Red clover is an alterative, expectorant, and antispasmodic.

Herb No. 9 (Schizandra)

This is the bonus herb. It is difficult to put together a combination of herbs to be a fundamental part of a Detox Regime without including the schizandra berry. So many toxins in our modern society are oxidizing agents. They range from chlorine in the water supply to the free radials that are generated as the result of so many reactions of toxic substances, both in the world at large and inside you. This is why *antioxidant* has become such a buzz word, and why the antioxidant nutrients such as vitamins A, C and E; and minerals such as selenium, zinc, and manganese (particularly selenium) have become so important.

You will recall that schizandra is an antioxidant and an antihepatotoxic, thus protecting that all-important liver. It is a tonic for the central nervous system, respiratory system, immune system, and uterus, and it improves lipid and carbohydrate metabolism. And in addition to protecting all these tissues, it gives a profound boost to your immune system. This one is built in to provide for your long-term health.

Herb No. 10 (Ginseng)

To round out the list, I have chosen ginseng — not because it is a Detox herb, although it does increase your immune function — but rather for the "feel-good factor." Ginseng is stomachic, antidepressive, immune stimulant, and tonic. It increases physical health and well-being and will give you an energy boost. As an antidepressant, it will also give you a mental boost, particularly if this is needed as a result of fatigue and lethargy.

Summary

- Herb No. 1 Gentian Root
- Herb No. 2 Milk Thistle
- Herb No. 3 Rhubarb Root
- Herb No. 4 Cat's Claw
- Herb No. 5 Poke Root
- Herb No. 6 Bucchu
- Herb No. 7 Coltsfoot
- Herb No. 8 Red Clover
- Herb No. 9 Schizandra
- Herb No. 10 Ginseng

Going on this Detox Regime and taking the Top Ten Tinctures will turn your health around and give you a new zest for life and living.

If you get the herbs in tincture form, you may choose to combine them all, in approximately equal proportions and then take two or three teaspoons of the mixture, in water, three times a day. This will provide you with less than the daily dose of each herb indicated in the herbal descriptions above. But this is intended. You are not specifically ill for one thing. Second, the actions of the herbs overlap, thus there is an interactive and cumulative effect when taking the combination.

Or, you may prefer to take them all separately. It is also possible that you will purchase some as tablets and, perhaps, some as combinations of two or more of them. That is fine.

For how long should you take the herbs? Take them for the first week anyway. If you started this program feeling as if you had no specific symptoms, you may not notice any specific changes, in which case you could then reduce the dose to once a day for the second week with a booster dose in weeks three and four. On the other hand, if you do feel really toxic, then I would suggest taking the mixture three times a day for the first week, twice a day for the second, and once a day for the last two weeks. After that, stop. Put them away and keep them in reserve for any time when you feel run down and toxic again. Remember that these are medicinal herbs, not nutritional herbs, particularly the first seven. Most of them should be saved for when you need them.

Maintenance

If you wish to maintain the progress you have made after the end of the four-week program, then you could plan to take a dose or two of the Top Ten herbal combination at intervals, when you feel the need. In spite of the above remark about medicinal herbs, it is true that you can safely go on drinking red clover tea and taking schizandra for long-term blood detoxing and antioxidant protection, and I would recommend this.

You should, of course, continue to incorporate all the culinary herbs and leaves in your diet and drink the various herbal teas, as appropriate to your needs, along with drinking dandelion coffee on a daily basis. Do this in conjunction with maintaining a good maintenance diet. Keeping your system clean and healthy is an ongoing process.

✢✢✢   ✢✢✢

✦ CHAPTER 17 ✦

Mini and Micro Detox Regimes

Mini Detox — for the Conservative Detoxer

If you really feel you are fairly healthy and do not want to take all the above ten herbs but would like a mini herbal Detox, then the following Regime is a possibility. However, I would not recommend this. If you feel you are in need of a Detox, I would encourage you to do the full Detox Regime. But, better than nothing, I would suggest that you follow the above regime of culinary herbs and the Detox Regime diet, and that you take this shortened list of herbs.

This is also an appropriate Detox Regime to follow if you have done the full program, some months have gone by, and you feel in need of a boost to get you back on track.

Step No. 1

Go through the descriptions in the Top Ten Tinctures list and incorporate all the culinary herbs and spices mentioned there in your cooking, salads and salad dressings.

Step No. 2

Add the various leaves such as nettle, nasturtium, and dandelion into your diet.

Step No. 3

Make sure that each day you drink the various herbal teas that were suggested: peppermint, rosehip, dandelion, etc., selecting those that are most appropriate to your needs.

Step No. 4

Take the following four herbs. This group will not, of course, give you as good or as profound a result as if you'd taken the full Top Ten Tinctures, but it is a feasible combination if you want to take a conservative approach. It will make a difference, particularly if you include all the other suggestions given about diet and lifestyle.

- Gentian root will help your upper digestive system.
- Dandelion will help your liver and lower digestive system and help to prevent constipation so that rhubarb root can be omitted. You will have to rely on its diuretic action instead of that of buchu.
- Cat's claw can be used for both your immune and lymphatic systems, so you can dispense with poke root.
- Red clover can do duty as an alterative, and can substitute for coltsfoot as an expectorant.

You cannot expect the results to be as good as if you had followed the full Top Ten program. If you are constipated — fewer than three soft and easy motions a day, and you probably are — then dandelion may need the support of generous servings of linseed or psyllium hulls to get things going when you omit rhubarb root.

Micro Detox — for the Lazy Detoxer

If you are daunted by the thought of either of the above Detox Regimes, or feel that you want some results but simply cannot be bothered to make huge changes or track down all the herbs, then you could consider the following program.

Step No. 1

Follow the diet recommended for Week One (see p.211). Do this for a full week, longer if possible, and then go to Week Four and plan how you will eat in the future, promising yourself that you will try to maintain this healthy lifestyle and not slip back into your old ways.

Step No. 2

Incorporate all the culinary herbs that are appropriate for your condition or situation.

Step No. 3

If you are only willing to take one medicinal herb, then golden seal is an obvious candidate.

It benefits all your mucous membranes, those lining the stomach, your lungs and bronchial tubes, and your urinary system and bladder. It is an expectorant and helps to expel mucus. It will boost your immune system and help you fight infections, and it will boost your lymphatic system and so facilitate the draining and removal of toxins from various parts of your body. In addition to all that, it will fight parasites, benefit the skin, and act as a tonic herb. It is thus an overall herb that will help you improve your health. Remember, however, that it is best not to take it if you are pregnant.

You should combine this with cups of dandelion coffee taken several times a day to support your liver, and take sufficient psyllium hulls or linseeds to prevent constipation.

Do not be lulled into a false sense of security, however. You will get out of this Regime in proportion to what you put in. While this Micro Detox Regime may lull you into thinking you have made the effort, that you have made some significant changes and that your health and overall well-being will improve dramatically, it won't. Small changes lead to small benefits.

However, this Micro Regime is a good one to use on a regular basis when you have broken all the rules. Go on it, for instance, if you have had a heavy weekend, woken up with a hangover and know you should not have stayed in that smoky atmosphere breathing all those fumes. Or take it after a week of heavy entertaining when you have overeaten and overdrunk, after the fun but unhealthy feasting of Christmas, or go on it two or three times a year after you have done an initial cleanout by doing the full Detox Regime.

+++   +++

+ CHAPTER 18 +

Experiment with Herbs

YOU MAY HAVE, AS WAS ASSUMED above, decided to follow a Detox Regime simply because you thought it was a good idea and to prevent, rather than treat, any particular symptoms. You may have done it because you felt generally toxic and lethargic, but without any specific health problems that you could put your finger on or name.

However, most people who are truly healthy generally feel they can take their health for granted. So it is highly probable that you have read this far and are thinking of starting on a Detox Regime because you have one or more specific problems.

With this in mind, you might want to work through the selection process again, paying attention to possible specific problems you may have. Any suggestions made here will only be a guide, of course. When it comes to the final selections, you will be doing this on the basis of your own specific needs.

If at any time you have doubts or questions about what you are doing, then you should consult a professional herbalist who can give you personalized advice. Keep in mind, too, that this is not a recommendation for a treatment protocol. The suggestions given here are simply ways of redirecting your Detox Regime toward your own particular needs. For treatment for specific conditions, you would be well advised to consult a professional.

It is also worth pointing out that there are, in fact, hundreds, if not thousands, of beneficial herbs. Different countries, different systems, and different people have their own preferences. You may have, know of, or have been advised to take a specific herb that has not been included here. If you wish to incorporate it into your Detox Regime, that is fine. Find out its specific roles, and then you will know where to put it in your choice, and for which herb you can use it as a substitute.

Herb Groups

Work through each of the sections, study the specific herbs in that Herbal Group. Instead of trying to select the best herb in each category, pick the herbs that incorporate in their action some of the other activities and benefits you are after.

You don't have to use an herb from each group. If your lungs are fine and you never get colds, but you do get indigestion, are constipated, and have skin problems, for instance, you could then focus on herbs for these problems (possibly adding more than one); and omit the herbs for lungs, catarrhal problem, or your immune system. If you do this, however, I would suggest that you consider including golden seal as a general herb and choose dandelion as your hepatic for its additional action as a diuretic.

Herb No. 1

My first choice for a sialogogue, to increase the flow of saliva and get your digestion off to a good start, was gentian root. However, the other possibilities discussed in that section include cayenne, ginger, licorice root, and thyme. While it is true that you can include cayenne, ginger, and thyme in your diet you may still want the added impetus of taking them in tincture format. You would choose cayenne or ginger as your sialogogue if you get frequent colds. You would choose licorice root if you have a lot of catarrh with wet bronchial coughs from time to time or if you are stressed; or your adrenal glands, the ones that pump out the stress hormones each time they are required, need help. Thyme would be your sialogogue of choice if you have reason to think you have parasites in your digestive tract or are asthmatic.

Gentian was also chosen for its action as a bitter, but the other possibilities were barberry, centaury, golden seal, and wormwood. It is already suggested that golden seal be included in the mixture, and you may feel that this is sufficient. Be warned, however, that many people are producing too little stomach acid without even knowing it or getting any specific symptoms, so it would be better to include a good bitter herb, at least at the start.

Barberry would be a good choice if you have gallstones or a gallbladder problem. Centaury would be a better choice if you are nervy and tense, or if you have a poor appetite; and wormwood would definitely be your choice if you think you have parasites in the gut, including worms.

You could choose either a sialagogue or a bitter herb. On the other hand, if your digestion is poor, then it would be worth including one of each.

Herb No. 2

Milk thistle was the original choice, but other herbs discussed include dandelion, greater celandine, balmony, barberry, black root, blue flag, boldo, fringe tree, vervain, wahoo, and yellow dock. The first three are excellent liver herbs, but the others could be more appropriate for you, depending on what specific problems you have. You should still, of course, drink dandelion coffee and eat the leaves.

Dandelion shares with milk thistle the advantage that it is readily available. Its main advantages over milk thistle are its roles as a diuretic and laxative. Greater celandine is an antispasmodic and useful if you get stomach or intestinal cramps. Balmony and barberry are anti-emetic, useful if you feel nauseated, at least until you have corrected the problem at the source. Blood root would be your choice if you have asthma and/or heart and circulation problems. Either blue flag or yellow dock would be a better choice if you have skin problems such as spots and pimples, acne, or eczema. They are both excellent general herbs for the skin, but as cholagogues, they also benefit your liver and help to prevent constipation. Boldo and fringe tree are useful if you have gallstones and suffer from cystitis. Vervain is helpful if you are nervy and tense or under a lot of stress and pressure, as it is a nervine, tonic, sedative, and anti-depressant, as well as being a hepatic. Wahoo is another herb that will help your circulation as well as supporting your liver.

Herb No. 3

The original choice for dealing with constipation and stimulating normal bowel function was rhubarb root. There are many other herbs you could choose for this purpose, including bog bean, elder, fringe tree, cascara, and senna.

Cascara and senna are both strong cathartics and should not be used on a regular basis, so I would not suggest that you build these into a combination remedy. However, if your constipation is severe, you could take one of the two once or twice until you get things moving more regularly. That leaves bog bean, elder, and fringe tree. Bog bean would be appropriate if you have rheumatism. Elder would be an excellent choice if you get frequent bouts of cold and flu. Fringe tree, like dandelion, is also a cholagogue and diuretic.

Herb No. 4

Our initial choice for your immune system was cat's claw, and that is still one of the best. However, some people may already have an individual preference for echinacea. While this is excellent for the immune system, it doesn't have so many other benefits as you will get from cat's claw.

Licorice could be your choice if your main immune problem is colds and flu plus catarrh and bronchial problems with a persistent cough, and if you are stressed. Myrrh and thyme are useful if you want to aim your immune activity at mouth and throat infections, though for this purpose they are best taken on their own as a mouthwash with which you can also gargle before swallowing them. Nasturtium is helpful if you are female and the infections you experience are commonly related to your reproductive organs — pelvic inflammatory disease, or uterine or vaginal infections.

Herb No. 5

Poke root was chosen for your lymphatic system. Alternatives include cleavers, golden seal, and wild indigo. Cleavers is an excellent herb if the lymphatic swelling and congestion involves the adenoids or tonsils, or if you suffer from psoriasis or cystitis. Golden seal has many other benefits to offer, as detailed above. Wild indigo is also an antimicrobial and one of the few febrifuges, so it helps to bring temperatures down safely and gently, and could be your choice if you get frequent or prolonged fevers.

Herb No. 6

Buchu was the chosen herb for your urinary system. Dandelion leaves, already suggested as a valuable part of your diet, will also act as a diuretic. So will the root when taken either as a tincture or as dandelion coffee. Boldo and couch grass are not only diuretics, but are useful demulcents for urinary infections and so are soothing, for instance, in cases of cystitis. Couch grass, in addition, is helpful if you also suffer from rheumatism.

Herb No. 7

For your lungs, the selection was coltsfoot. There are several others you could choose: comfrey, daisy, elecampane, grindelia, horehound, linseed, lobelia, mullein, pleurisy root, poke root, red clover, and thuja.

Comfrey is an astringent, demulcent, and vulnerary as well as being an expectorant, and useful if there is internal bleeding or healing is required. Daisy is also an astringent and bitter, so it's useful if your other main problem is with indigestion. Elecampane or linseed would be a good choice if you get frequent coughs; and lobelia would be your choice if these coughs are deep-seated, with phlegm that simply won't come up or if you are asthmatic. Grindelia should be your choice if you have low blood pressure. Horehound is also an antispasmodic and helpful if you get a tight chest or have a tendency to be asthmatic. Mullein offers the added benefit of being a mild sedative. Pleurisy root is another antispasmodic and will help to improve your digestion. Red clover would be a good choice if you also have skin problems. Thuja is useful if your cough is dry rather than phlegmy and has been going on for some time. And poke root may already be your choice, as discussed for Herb No 5.

Herb No. 8

The herb chosen for your skin was red clover. Other suggestions were too many to go through here. However, four of the main ones you could consider in place of red clover are blue flag, burdock, cleavers, and yellow dock. Blue flag will also benefit your liver and colon. Burdock is particularly useful it you suffer from eczema and is a useful diuretic. Cleavers also benefits the lymphatic system. Yellow dock is useful if you have acne or psoriasis, as are sarsparilla and sassafras. Figwort deserves a mention and is helpful as it can help your heart. Read through the others, and choose the one that best suits your own particular needs.

Herbs No. 9 and 10

I offered no choice here. I do think that schizandra should stay on your list for the reasons mentioned in the discussion on that herb. Ginseng you can leave out, particularly if you have plenty of energy, but it is a useful herb to include if you are tired.

Summary

So there you have it. You can use the functions summary in Table i at the end of the book for quick reference. You are now in a position to select the herbs you want, according to your own particular needs. Have the courage to experiment. The range included here will also give you the opportunity to try these alternatives if your first herb of choice is not easy to find.

Whatever you do, come clean. So many health problems and so much personal misery can be avoided if you create a healthy, low-toxin lifestyle. Some of the changes called for may seem radical to you, yet I can assure you that you can live well and have fun and *still* be healthy if you set your mind to it. Instead of saying to yourself, "I'd love to have/eat/drink so-and-so, but I can't/mustn't/it isn't permitted"; say instead, "I don't want to have/eat/drink so-and-so, I don't want what they would do to me." By choosing to focus on avoiding the harm that things can do to you rather than focusing on feeling deprived because of the perceived pleasures of a particular habit, you can soon come to prefer your new and healthier choices.

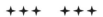

PART VI

Where to Find Herbs

✦ CHAPTER 19 ✦

Detox from the Kitchen

THIS CHAPTER IS FOR THOSE PEOPLE who like the idea of using herbs; who want to clean up their act; who would like to feel healthier, more energetic, more clear-headed, and be slim, but who stop short at the thought of taking herbs too seriously.

It is also for those people who live some distance from stores or outlets that sell medicinal herbs. While it is true that almost all of them can be bought by mail order or via the Web, it is also true that some people do not like to shop in this fashion.

So in this chapter I have included all the herbs that can, generally, be found in your local supermarket or health-food store. These are the herbs or spices you could expect to find in a well-stocked kitchen, either for seasoning food or for use as herbal teas.

You will find a list of the relevant herbs with a brief description of where to find them, an explanation of what they do, and suggestions as to how they can be used. For those with a more significant medical use, such as garlic and peppermint, you will find a more comprehensive description in Part IV.

You will find that the majority of these herbs are beneficial to your digestive system, and it is interesting to wonder at their use. Is it possible that, over the centuries, people found that the addition of these herbs not only provided flavor but aided digestion as well? I think it is. Some of them have a range of other benefits as well, so look out for these, and particularly the ones relevant to any problems you may have, as you read through them.

Allspice

Pimenta Officinalis gets its name from the fact that it tastes somewhat like a combination of several spices, principally nutmeg, cinnamon, and cloves. It is generally available on the spice shelves and is used in pickles and chutneys. Try adding some the next time you are cooking red cabbage. It is an aromatic, carminative, and digestive stimulant. It will help to tone up your digestive system and to relieve bloating and flatulence.

Aloe Vera

This has already been discussed (p.192). It is readily available either as the juice (for drinking) or the gel (for topical application) from most health-food stores and some supermarkets. One or two glasses a day can easily be incorporated into your daily routine.

Aniseed

Pimpinella anisum is generally available on the spice shelves. It is aromatic, antispasmodic, carminative, expectorant, and parasiticide. So it too will help to relieve flatulence and bloating; it will also help to kill off some of the unwanted pathogens in your digestive tract and to help clear unwanted mucus from your throat and lungs. It gives an interesting flavor to desserts or pastries but be wary of using this as an excuse to have too many sugar-rich foods. Try incorporating these seeds into the sauce next time you cook fish. The seeds can also be nibbled after a meal.

Basil

Ocimum basilicum is available on the dried herb shelves. You will also find it, commonly, among the fresh herbs in the vegetable section, either already cut or as a small grow-pot. It is antispasmodic, digestive stimulant, and carminative. It has been found to be useful in the treatment of stomach cramps, gastric catarrh, flatulence, and bloating, and of abdominal cramps or irritable bowel syndrome. Use it generously in tomato dishes. Layer the leaves between layers of sliced fresh tomatoes, drizzle olive oil over it, and you have an immediate, tasty, and cleansing salad. If you cook with it, it is best to add it to the dish at the last minute, or its flavor is inclined to get lost.

PESTO

The main ingredient of this Genoese addition to Italian cooking is basil. Essentially it is a combination of crushed garlic, finely chopped basil, parmesan cheese, and olive oil. The exact proportions are up to you, but a starting guide would be three cloves of garlic and five tablespoons of finely chopped basil. These should be pounded together in a pestle and mortar, if you have one. If not, put the basil in a food processor, and add the garlic squeezed through a garlic press and blend. Add about one cup of grated parmesan cheese and sufficient olive oil to make a smooth paste, probably about two or three tablespoons, and blend well together.

This can be served with pasta or put, instead of a pat of butter, on grilled fish.

Add a couple of tablespoons of pine nuts for a subtle new flavor.

Pesto variations

These variations do not come from Genoa, but there is nothing to stop you from using a wide range of herbs instead of basil. It is delicious, for instance, made from fresh coriander leaves. For vegans, the parmesan cheese can be replaced by some of the soy or rice cheeses that are available, or by adding ground sunflower seeds or walnuts.

Bay

Laurus nobilis produces firm leaves an inch or two long. You will generally find them, whole or crushed, on the dried herb shelves. It is astringent, aromatic, digestive, and stomachic. Its main use is for the digestive system, to stimulate its normal function and prevent problems. Some people find that the whole herb is the easiest to use. They put it whole into a range of cooked dishes to add flavor and then put it to one side. To get the full benefit, however, it should be crushed into a fine powder and eaten with the meal.

Cardamom

Elettaria cardamomum is available as seeds on the spice shelves. It is carminative, sialagogue, and aromatic, so will both stimulate digestion and relieve flatulence and bloating. It is commonly added to curries. Add it to pastry for an interesting flavor, or chew the seeds after a meal.

CARDAMOM APERITIF

Add some cardamom seeds to a bottle of sherry and allow them to steep for a few days. Drinking this before a meal will help reduce any tendency toward flatulence.

Caraway

Carum carvi is available as seeds on the herb shelves. It is anti-spasmodic, astringent, carminative, expectorant, aromatic, emmenogogue, and galactogogue. It is traditionally added to cabbage dishes, possibly with the aim of reducing the flatulence this vegetable can cause in some people.

Cayenne

This has been discussed (p.86). You will find it on the spice shelves and can enjoy it any time you choose a curry. Not only is it a strong sialagogue and a carminative, thus stimulating the flow of digestive juices and helping to relieve flatulence, it is also a tonic and an antiseptic. It will, if you recall the recipe for "Kick-a-germ-joy-juices" help to relieve the symptoms of the common cold or a bout of the flu and speed your recovery.

Celery

Apium graveolens can be found on the fresh vegetable shelves, but it can also be found as a seed on the herb rack. The seeds are carminative, and so will help your digestion, but this is an herb with other uses. It is antirheumatic, and its main use is in the treatment of arthritis, rheumatism, and gout. It is diuretic, and so will help your Detox Regime by encouraging the elimination of toxins in the urine.

CELERY SALAD

You may be saying, "But I use celery already in my salads." That may be so, but you probably don't use the seeds, and it is these that are particularly carminative. Make your salad in the usual way, toss with your chosen dressing, and then sprinkle the celery seeds on top. If you frequently suffer from flatulence, then make a habit of having a side salad with meals and sprinkling the salad with these seeds.

Chamomile

This comes in two forms, both of them *Compositae.* English chamomile is *Anthemus nobile,* and German chamomile is *Matricaria chamomilla.* Chamomile is generally available in the form of an herb tea, and the flower heads are used. English chamomile is anodyne, antispasmodic, aromatic, bitter, tonic, stimulant, and stomachic. German chamomile is antispasmodic, antiinflammatory, carminative, analgesic, antiseptic, and vulnerary.

Chamomile can be drunk as a relaxing herb tea at the end of a meal. It will help to settle the digestion and is sufficiently gentle to be drunk by babies. Pour the cooled tea into a bottle, and give it to them as a remedy for colic.

It can also be used externally. Use wet teabags as eye pads for sore or inflamed eyes. Use it as a wash on skin infections, first as an antiseptic, and then for its antiinflammatory and healing properties.

Chervil

Anthriscus cerefolium can sometimes be found among the dried herbs. It is a digestive stimulant, helping to normalize your digestion.

It is also useful in a Detox Regime, as it is both a diuretic and an expectorant. Add it to a variety of savory dishes, both meat and vegetables, and to salads.

CHERVIL SOUP

Melt two tablespoons of butter in a pan. Chop 8 cups of chervil leaves and add to the butter. Add a teaspoon of dried tarragon and another of dried chervil. Put the lid on, and simmer the mixture for 15 minutes. Add 4½ cups of stock and simmer for another 15 minutes. Put 2 egg yolks in a bowl, and whisk with a fork. Slowly add 4½ cups of the soup, then add this mixture to the remaining stock, stir and serve with a scoop of natural yogurt in the center.

CHERVIL-TOSSED VEGETABLES

You can spice up a relatively mild-tasting vegetable by tossing it, once cooked, with a handful of chopped fresh chervil leaves. Lightly cook a vegetable such as sliced zucchini or diced marrow, drain, add a small amount of olive oil and the freshly chopped chervil, squeeze over some lemon juice, and serve. If you want the flavor of lemon without the bitterness, add chopped fresh lemon balm instead of the lemon juice.

Chives

Allium schoenoprasum is commonly available as bunches of the fresh leaves. They are also available dried and chopped, in packets. You may get a small, potted plant of it, in which case cut the leaves, as you want them, an inch or two above the base, and they will regrow to provide you with more.

Chives are aromatic and a useful digestive aid.

CHIVES IN COOKING

Anytime you would like the flavor of onions but would like to be mild, choose chives. Later you will find a recipe for Mint Cheese (p.252). You can do the same thing with chives. Be generous.

Cut a large bunch of chives into ¼-inch lengths and sprinkle generously over a salad or steamed vegetables.

Lay a bed of chives in a casserole dish, place the fish on top, pour on some white wine, and bake in a moderate oven.

For an unusual salad, interlayer slices of finely cut orange with layers of thinly sliced red onions (try it before you reel back in disbelief), and sprinkle chopped chives on top.

Stuff red or green peppers with brown rice combined with a generous handful of chopped chives and crushed garlic.

Cinnamon

Cinnamomum zeylanicum is available in the spice section. It generally comes in two forms. The rolled and dried inner bark of the shoots may be available in pieces, or as the ground powder. Cinnamon is an aromatic, astringent, carminative, and stimulant. Thus it will help to tighten up the tissues, relieve flatulence, and give you a pep-up.

Cloves

Eugenia caryophyllus are one of the more common spices. If you don't find it, look on the baking shelves. It is an aromatic, carminative, and stimulant and so good for your digestive system. Traditionally it is used as an analgesic for toothaches.

Coriander (Cilantro)

Coriandrum sativum is a spice commonly used in Indian cooking. You will find the seeds, whole or ground, on the spice shelves. You will also find the fresh leaves, either cut and sold in a bunch, or as a small potted plant, available in the fresh vegetable section. It is an aromatic carminative and very good for your digestion.

CORIANDER SALAD

Chop two medium-sized onions into small pieces. Add four tablespoons of chopped fresh coriander leaves and two tablespoons of freshly squeezed lemon juice. If you want the flavor of lemon without the sourness, omit some of the lemon juice and add chopped fresh leaves of lemon balm. Serve on a bed of green leaves.

SPICY CORIANDER SALAD

Proceed as above, but add two tomatoes, chopped; one tablespoon of grated fresh ginger root; a red chili pepper chopped, with the seeds removed. (Remove the seeds with a teaspoon, not your fingers, otherwise future contact with any broken or delicate skin, such as your eyes, can be extremely painful.) Serve on a bed of lettuce.

Corn Silk

Zea mays may seem to be an unusual inclusion here. However, if you find fresh corn cobs on the vegetable shelves, with the green tassel still hanging out from between the leaves, don't ignore it. The fresh green tassel, or "silk," is an excellent herb for your kidneys. It is a diuretic, demulcent tonic and will help to encourage the loss of toxins in the urine. Simply chop it up and eat it with the rest of the vegetable, or pour boiling water on it and make an infusion or tea.

Cucumber

Cucumis sativus is normally thought of as a vegetable to be served either in salads or sometimes cooked, with poached salmon. The seeds are usually discarded. This is a shame, as they can offer several benefits. The fruit and seeds are demulcent, soothing to the mucous membranes; diuretic; so helpful in fluid retention; and aperient, helping to prevent constipation. It is also a vulnerary; try using slices of cucumber as eye pads. You will find that they are very soothing. Cucumber is found in a number of herbal cosmetics and toiletries for this reason.

The seeds are anthelmintic and so should be eaten, not discarded, if you think you have worms or similar parasites. Even if you don't have them, the seeds can be a useful prophylactic. It has also been suggested that cucumber can help to dissolve uric acid and so reduce the risk of kidney stones and gout.

CUCUMBER AND SALMON

It is easy to think of cucumber solely as a minor component of a salad, but try this idea next time you cook salmon.

Allow one long cucumber for two people. Peel it and cut it in half lengthways so you can scoop out the seeds and juice in the center. Save the seeds. Then slice it as thinly as you possibly can. Spread the slices over a large surface, either a large platter or a tray that can handle getting wet. Sprinkle the cucumber with salt, tilt the platter, and allow the juices that come out to drain away. After an hour or two, drain off all the liquid, pressing the cucumber to squeeze out as much as possible. Mix a few teaspoons of apple cider vinegar with the compressed cucumber, and serve with poached salmon and new potatoes, decorated with sprigs of fresh dill.

Dry the seeds, and nibble on them to ease any indigestion.

Cumin

Cuminum cyminum is available as the whole or ground seed on most spice shelves and is used extensively in curries. It is an antispasmodic, carminative, stimulant, and so helpful if you suffer from flatulence and bloating or from stomach or abdominal cramps.

Dill

Anethum graveolens is available as the seed, either whole or ground, on the spice shelves, and also as the dried leaves. If you are lucky, you may even find some fresh leaves for sale among the vegetables. It is antispasmodic, carminative, and stomachic — so good for your digestion.

DILLED CARROTS

Fresh dill has a wonderful flavor. Pour a tablespoon of fresh yogurt over a dish of lightly steamed fresh carrots. Then sprinkle chopped fresh dill leaves over the top. Delicious.

Fennel

Foeniculum vulgare is available as a seed on the herb shelves. It is also available as a vegetable; however, the leaves and seeds of this are less useful than the herbal form. The latter grows with a very small root, putting all its energy into growing the long stems and graceful leaves. It is aromatic, antispasmodic, carminative, diuretic, stimulant, galactagogue, expectorant, and rubefacient.

It is an excellent stomachic and helps to ensure proper digestive function. This is another tasty herb to chew at the end of a meal. It helps to relieve colic and flatulence. As a diuretic, it encourages the flow of urine and the loss of toxins via the kidneys.

In addition, it helps to encourage the flow of breast milk. It is calming and soothing to the lungs and bronchial tubes; as an expectorant it helps to expel unwanted mucus, and it is used in the treatment of coughs and bronchitis. Use it as a gargle, and then swallow to get the rest of the benefits.

The herb can be used externally on muscular pains and rheumatism and as eye pads for the treatment of problems such as conjunctivitis, and inflamed eyelids.

Fenugreek

Trigonella foenum-graecum has an unusual three-dimensionally shaped seed. It is available in the spice racks and used in curries. Fenugreek is a mucilaginous demulcent, expectorant, galactagogue, and tonic. Unlike previous herbs, it is not of primary use in the digestive tract, although it is a mild bitters. Because of its demulcent action, is gentle on the digestive tract. Instead, it is a useful expectorant and helpful for sore throats. Gargle with it and then swallow. Add it to a curry the next time you cook one.

It can be used externally on wounds, cuts, boils, and other skin problems.

Flax (Linseed)

Linum usitatissumum is usually available as linseed, from health food stores. We have already discussed it for the digestive tract and to prevent constipation, for lung problems and for external use on skin problems. You will probably have it in your cupboard anyway so add it to foods for all these benefits.

Garlic

Allium sativum has been fully discussed in previous sections. Use it extensively in cooking and add it to salad dressings.

GARLIC SOUP

Mince six large cloves of garlic and cook gently in two tablespoons of butter. Do not let it brown. Sprinkle in a tablespoon of wholemeal flour, mix thoroughly and then gradually blend in 4½ cups of stock and bring to the boil. Add two bay leaves, a pinch of mace powder, season with freshly-ground black pepper and salt, simmer for 15 minutes, and serve, decorated with fresh coriander leaves.

Ginger

Zingiber officinale has been fully discussed already (p.88). You can buy it as the fresh root from the vegetable section or in powdered form from the spice section. Use it generously in cooking, or pour boiling water on it to make a refreshing drink.

Ginseng

Panax ginseng is commonly available from health-food stores as tablets or capsules or in the form of an herb tea. It is antidepressive, demulcent, stomachic, and a stimulant. It is of only modest use for detoxing but will certainly give you an important energy boost.

Horseradish

Armoracia rusticana — the root is commonly available, already processed and served up as horseradish sauce, with beef and other red meats. It is a carminative, diuretic, mild laxative, and stimulant.

It is useful as an aid to the immune system in the treatment of colds and fevers. As a carminative, it helps the digestive system, particularly after a large meal such as the traditional Sunday roast beef. It will help to ease those potential cramping pains as you relax afterwards, regretting that second helping. As a diuretic, it has been used as an aid to the kidneys and to increase the flow of urine.

A very simple horseradish sauce can be made by grating horseradish and adding it to mayonnaise. If you feel slightly more ambitious, try the recipe below.

HORSERADISH SAUCE

Grate horseradish until you have four tablespoons of the herb. Add ½ cup of Greek-style natural yogurt and a dash of freshly squeezed lemon juice. Season with salt and freshly ground black pepper.

If you prefer to have it creamier but don't want to use cream, add a small amount of olive oil.

To achieve a somewhat more gentle flavor, add some cooked and puréed cooking apples.

Irish Moss

Chondrus crispus is fairly readily available from health-food stores. It has been mentioned earlier (p.196) and can be converted into an infusion by pouring boiling water on it. It is useful for both your digestive system and for bronchial infections.

Juniper Berries

Juniperus communis has dried ripe berries that can sometimes be found on the herb shelves. They were discussed in the section on your kidneys. They can be made into a drink by infusing them in boiling water.

Kelp

This is not, strictly speaking, an herb, but neither is Irish moss. Kelp is a form of dried seaweed. It usually comes loose as either powder, granules, or tablets, all available from your local health-food store. It is a rich source of iodine and other trace minerals and can help to stimulate and tone up your whole metabolism. This benefits your energy and your well-being, as well as your capacity to Detox successfully and safely.

Lemon Grass

Cymbopogon citrates can often be bought fresh from the vegetable section of your local supermarket. It makes a refreshing tea when boiling water is poured on it, or adds a delicate lemon flavor to savory dishes, without the sourness of fresh lemon juice. It is refreshing and a mild stomachic.

Marjoram

Marjorana hortensis, or sweet marjoram, is a readily available culinary herb. See *oregano* for more information.

Mustard

Brassica alba and *Brassica nigra* are familiar to most people. Use the English form, either as a powder or already made into a paste by the addition of water. It is a diuretic, emetic, irritant, rubefacient, and stimulant.

Nutmeg

Myristica fragrans is a common spice. It can be bought in the powdered form or as the large, round and brown seed, ready for grating. It is an aromatic, carminative, hallucinogenic, and stimulant. It helps digestion and reduces wind and flatulence, but should only be taken in small quantities to avoid the hallucinogenic effects.

SPICED PUMPKIN SOUP

Cook pumpkin soup in the usual way, but add a pinch of nutmeg to it for a deliciously different flavor and as an aid to digestion.

Oregano

Origanum vulgare, also known as wild marjoram, is readily available as the dried herb. It can also sometimes be bought as the fresh herb, in bunches. It is an antiseptic, expectorant, emmenagogue, and rubefacient. It will help to clear your lungs and reduce a fever.

Use it as a mouthwash for the treatment of local infections, or gargle with it for a sore or infected throat. It is also helpful as a tea; or added to food for the treatment of headaches.

OREGANO AND PARSLEY SAUCE WITH TOMATO

This is another great way to use a lot of herbs to make a tasty sauce to serve with pasta or meat dishes. Warm one tablespoon of olive oil. Crush three cloves of garlic and add to the oil but do not allow it to brown. Chop and add four tomatoes and cook until they are just soft. Finally, add one tablespoon each of finely chopped fresh oregano and parsley. Cook for another five minutes, season to taste, and serve.

Parsley

Petroselinum crispum is probably our most common culinary herb. The leaves can be bought fresh or dried. They are carminative, diuretic, expectorant, and emmenagogue. Use parsley generously in sauces and as a seasoning. Not only does it add flavor but it aids digestion. It is a rich source of vitamin C and iron, and as a good diuretic, is a useful cleanser.

EASY PARSLEY SAUCE

I have never understood why so much effort is put into making a white sauce in, what seems to me, the most difficult way possible. Following the various Cordon Bleu methods and making a variety of roués, I frequently produced something that looked like lumpy porridge that had to be poured through a sieve before it could be served. Now I do it the easy way.

Put one cup of liquid, cold, in a saucepan. The liquid can be anything from water or stock, or any kind of milk (soy or cow's). Personally I rely on the milk my own goats' produce, but that is not possible for everyone. Then add two tablespoons of flour; this can be wheat flour, but barley flour makes a good alternative, and ¼ cup of olive oil. Stir briskly, bring to a boil, and allow to simmer for about ten minutes or until it has both thickened and cooked. Taste it — you will soon know.

Then add your herbs. If you are using parsley, you can hardly use too much. My aunt used to use so much that it had to be chopped up in the food processor in several batches, and the sauce was dark green and ridged with the stuff. As she used to say, served this way it was another vegetable in itself.

The other classical use of parsley is as parsley salad, otherwise known as tabouleh. This is a dish from the Middle East and comes in a variety of forms. When made badly, it is a fairly tasteless dish of cracked wheat with a few herbs through it. At its best, it is a flavorful dish of finely chopped parsley into which is added a small amount of cracked grains and a few chopped vegetables.

TABOULEH

Put three cups of cracked or crushed wheat in a bowl, pour on sufficient cold water to cover it, and allow to stand until the wheat has softened. Strain it and squeeze to remove excess water. Add double this volume of finely chopped parsley, three tablespoons each of chopped lemon balm and mint, half a cup of chopped chives, and one ripe tomato, chopped. Make sure the result looks like an enticing dark green dish of parsley, with additions. If it does not, then add more parsley.

Then it is time for the dressing. This is a combination of olive oil and lemon juice. Just as you would do for any other salad, combine the two in a ratio of approximately three to one, and use sufficient to lightly coat the ingredients. Season with black pepper.

If you are allergic to wheat, the crushed wheat can be replaced with a similar amount of either cooked brown rice or cooked buckwheat (unrelated to wheat itself). Although the result is slightly different, it can be just as delicious.

Peppermint

Mentha piperita is one of the best carminatives and was discussed in the section on flatulence. It is generally available as an herb tea and makes an excellent drink to have after a heavy meal or when you have a cold. It should not be confused with its relative, spearmint.

Spearmint

Mentha spicata is an antispasmodic, carminative, stomachic, though less so than peppermint and is a mild diuretic. This is the mint usually made into mint sauce and served with lamb. Here is another delicious way to serve it.

MINTED SOFT CHEESE

For this, you can use any type of soft cheese you like: ricotta cheese, cottage cheese, or cream cheese. I make it with the curd I make from my goats' milk at the stage where I would otherwise press it into a hard cheese.

Collect a huge bunch of fresh mint. Strip the leaves from the stems and chop finely. It works best if you nearly purée the leaves in a food processor. Combine this with the soft cheese. The proportions are really up to you. Season to taste.

You can include other herbs as well, such as crushed garlic or ground celery seeds, and make this with any other combinations of herbs of your choice. It is an excellent and enjoyable way of adding a wide range of herbs to your diet in considerable quantities.

Serve with salad, lightly steamed or stir-fried vegetables, or any other way that suits you.

Pimento

See Allspice.

Pumpkin

Cucurbita pepo — The seeds have already been mentioned as an anthelmantic (p.119). They can be bought from most health-food stores and eaten plain or added to stir-fry dishes or salads.

Serve them up as snacks to enjoy before a meal while you are having a carminative aperitif.

A CARMINATIVE APERITIF

You can, of course, use any form of alcohol for this, but it works well with sherry or white wines. Choose the seeds of any of the carminative herbs in the table on page 57, add them to your chosen alcohol, and allow to steep. If you use wine, you must drink it fairly soon or the wine will oxidize. If you choose sherry, you can allow if to stand almost indefinitely. The following are delicious: aniseed, caraway, cumin, cardamom, coriander, and dill. You can also soak slivers of ginger in the sherry and make your own equivalent of ginger wine. Equally, you can simply add to the efforts of others and add even more juniper berries to your bottle of gin.

Quassia

Picrasma excelsor is sometimes available among the spices. It is used in Asian cooking; should not be confused with cinnamon bark; and is anthelmintic, bitter, sialogogue, and tonic, so it can contribute in several ways to a Detox Regime.

Rosehips

Rosa canina is generally available as an herbal tea. The fruits and seeds of the dog rose are mildly astringent, diuretic, and laxative. Drink it as a refreshing tea and to help clean out your digestive system and kidneys.

Rosemary

Rosmarinus officinalis — the leaves are commonly available on herb shelves. They are aromatic, antispasmodic, antidepressive, antiseptic, carminative, parasiticide, and rubefacient. This is another herb that helps to improve your digestion and eliminate parasites and has a variety of other uses.

Saffron

Crocus sativus, the real thing, is usually available as the thin red filaments or stigmas. It is expensive, and substitutes are often sold in its place. Look out for the real thing. It is anodyne, antispasmodic, aphrodisiac, emmenogogue, expectorant, and sedative.

Sage

Salvia officinalis is one of the more common culinary herbs, usually thought of, in combination with thyme, as an herb to use when stuffing the turkey. It is antiseptic, astringent, antispasmodic, carminative, and aids digestion.

Tarragon

Artemisia dracunculus is a much underrated herb with a delicious flavor. If you are growing it, start with a plant rather than the seeds. It is diuretic and stomachic and so helpful in a Detox Regime.

Turmeric

Curcuma longal is a yellow-colored powder used in curries. It is a rich antioxidant, its main benefit, and is a mild aromatic and stimulant. Add it generously, in tablespoon quantities, to a curry next time you make one.

Thyme

See p.89.

Valerian

Valeriana officinalis is commonly available as an herbal tea. It is antispasmodic, carminative, hypnotic, hypotensive, and sedative.

It is generally used to help you relax and sleep well, but has also helped to relieve cramps and intestinal colic.

So, from this you can see that almost all the herbs and spices you might use in cooking have some beneficial effect. Insofar as they nearly all act on and improve the state of your digestive system, they have a contribution to make to your Detox Regime, for we know that is important.

Their action may not always be as strong as that of some of the medicinal herbs, but when you use them both generously and judiciously their combined contribution can be significant.

Get into the habit of using herbs regularly, both in cooking and as herbal teas. They are often even more delicious when fresh. Most of them can be grown in either a small corner of your garden or in pots, either on a patio or terrace or indoors.

HERBAL RISOTTO

An excellent way to incorporate a large quantity of herbs into your diet is to make this flavorful risotto.

For four people, cook one cup of brown rice until it is just tender and then drain. While the rice is cooking, sauté a finely chopped onion in one tablespoon of olive oil, add two cloves of garlic, crushed, and — be brave now — one whole cup of fresh herbs, finely chopped. Make your own selection. You have learned a lot about the most common culinary herbs; the next chapter will tell you a lot about other herbs you can grow in your garden. Choose the ones that both offer the medicinal actions you want and that please your palate. Finally, add two tablespoons of pine nuts, or pumpkin or sunflower seeds.

This can be served hot or cold. Because it has a rich flavor of its own, it is best served with a simple meat dish and some steamed vegetables such as carrots or cauliflower.

✦✦✦ ✦✦✦

+ CHAPTER 20 +

Detox from the Garden

THERE ARE MANY USEFUL HERBS that are not available from the supermarkets, but readily available from garden centers and seed suppliers. If you are an enthusiastic gardener, you may already be growing them, or have them cropping up in unexpected places. Even if you are not a keen gardener, you may have a garden space and be interested in experimenting. A helpful book you could consult is *Food for Free* by Richard Mabey. He shows you the plants that may very well be growing in your garden, which can be introduced to your diet.

Herbs come in all shapes and sizes. If you do not already have an elm tree, it may be a while before you can harvest your own slippery elm powder, but there is nothing to stop you planting some of the medicinal herbs and getting a harvest in a few months' time — or even less in the case of some quick-growing herbs and depending on the time of year when you start.

No garden? Relax. You can grow an amazing number of herbs in pots on windowsills, or indoors where there is good daylight. On the next page, I have listed some of the herbs that are readily available, either as plants or as seeds, from garden centres and gardening catalogs.

To avoid repetition, I have, in most cases, simply stated their actions; many of them have already been covered in some detail. The use you can make of the others will, by now, be obvious to you from their extended description.

Inherent in the concept of this chapter is the fact that you will be growing these herbs for yourself, so in most instances you will be making the flowers and leaves into an infusion or tea. The general quantities are one to two teaspoons per cup, but you can adjust the amount to suit your taste. For some other herbs, such as soapwort, the root is used and specific instructions are given.

Agrimony

Agrimonia eupatoria grows wild in hedgerows, but is less common in cooler regions. It is an astringent, diuretic tonic, and has been used successfully in the treatment of jaundice.

Alexanders

Available in seed catalogs under this name, it is also known as black lovage. *Smyrnium olisatrum* looks somewhat like wild angelica. It is should not be confused with lovage or *Levisticum officinale*. It is used for indigestion, colic, flatulence and fevers.

Alfalfa

Medicago sativa, also known as buffalo herb or lucerne, is a diuretic and tonic. The leaves can be drunk as a tea and are alkalizing, mineral-rich, and have been recommended for people suffering from arthritis. Eat the sprouts with salad.

Angelica

See p.151.

Aniseed

See p.237.

Arnica

Arnica montana is well known as an herb to use externally on bruises, sprains, and other wounds, to any areas that have suffered from physical trauma. It can also be used on chilblains provided the skin is unbroken. It is used internally in homoeopathic form, but is rarely taken internally as an herbal preparation.

Basil

See p.237.

Bearberry

See p.168.

Bistort

Polygonum bistorta is an extremely strong astringent and an alterative and diuretic. It contains up to 20 percent tannins. As an astringent, a decoction made from the root is used externally for sores and to reduce bleeding, and is used as a mouthwash for inflammation of the mouth in general and for gum problems. It is effective in the treatment of diarrhea, even when severe and accompanied by bleeding, and is useful in all conditions of bleeding, internal and external. As an alterative, it is a good blood cleanser.

Borage

Borago officinalis is a diuretic, demulcent, and emolient. It is useful in the treatment of fevers, particularly in relation to the lungs.

Broom

The young tips of the flowering branches of *Cytisus scoparius* should be collected in spring and early summer. They are diuretic and cathartic.

Burdock

See p.184.

Burnet

Sanguisorba officinalis is an astringent and tonic. The venerable herbalist Culpeper said of it, "This is an herb the Sun challenges dominion over, and is a most precious herb, little inferior to Betony, the continual use of it preserves the body in health and the spirits in vinegar." Three or four sprigs of it in a glass of red wine were thought to do the trick. The flavor is reminiscent of cucumber.

- Make an infusion from the fresh or dried leaves or add to salads.

Caraway

See p.239.

Catnip

See p.152.

Centaury

See p.91.

Chamomile

See p.240.

Chervil

See p.240

Chickweed

See p.194.

Chives

See p.241.

Clary Sage

See sage, p.254. Clary sage has similar uses but a slightly different flavor.

Cleavers

See p.158.

Coltsfoot

See p.175.

Comfrey

See p.176 and 195.

Coneflower

Available from nurseries as seeds, coneflower is, in fact, another name for echinacea. See p.141.

Coriander (Cilantro)

See p.242.

Cumin

See p.244.

Daisy

See p.177.

Dandelion

See p.111, 125, and 165.

Dill

See p.244.

Echinacea

See p.141.

Elecampane

See p.177.

Epazote, Wormseed

This is another herb often known by its Latin or homoeopathic name, *Chenopodium ambrosioides*. Like wormwood, with which it should not be confused, it is an anthelmintic, and useful if you think you have intestinal parasites. It is effective against round-worms and hookworms but not against tapeworms. As the name implies, it is the seed, more specifically the oil from the seed, that is particularly effective.

Evening Primrose

You will probably not be surprised to learn that it is the oil found in the seed of evening primrose, or *Oenothera biennis*, that is particularly valuable.

Fat Hen

Fat hen or Good King Henry, *Chenopodium bonus, Henricus*, is a useful vegetable and can stand in for spinach in any dish you choose to prepare. As a perennial, it will stay loyal and come up year after year with no extra effort from you.

Fennel

See p.245.

Feverfew

Chrysanthemum parthenium is aperient, carminative, bitter, and emmenagogue. It is useful in the treatment of nervous tension, hence its use in the treatment of migraine headaches. It is also a general tonic.

Fuller's Teasel

Also sometimes known as Fuller's herb, this is soapwort (See p.272).

Garlic

See p.143.

Gentian

See p.92.

Gipsywort

Lycopus europaeus is an astringent and sedative.

Goat's Beard

Tragopogon pratensis was used extensively in medieval times but is rarely used today as a medicinal herb. The roots were eaten as a vegetable; the stems were treated as we now treat asparagus. A decoction of the root was used to treat indigestion and "disorders of the liver."

Goat's Rue

Galega officinalis, a legume, is a diaphoretic, diuretic, and galactogogue. An infusion of the fresh plant is said to be soothing to tired feet.

Gravelroot

Eupatorium purpureum is a diuretic and nervine and, as its common name implies, useful in the treatment of urinary gravel and chronic kidney problems. It has also been used in the treatment of gout and rheumatism.

Greater Celandine

See p.129.

Grindelia

See p.178.

Heartsease

Viola tricolor, also known as wild pansy, was traditionally used as a remedy for epilepsy and asthma, and the flowers were thought, as you might guess, to benefit the heart.

Heliotrope

Heliotrope, or in the Latin form *Heliotropium peruviana*, is given that name name from the fact that it follows the sun's path throughout the day and at night turns its face back to the east to repeat the process the next day. It is used mainly as a homoeopathic remedy in the treatment of sore throats.

Henbane

Hyoscyamus niger comes from the same order as potatoes, tomatoes, and tobacco. It is anodyne, antispasmodic, and calmative and was used by the Greeks and Romans to reduce pain. However, it is also a potentially poisonous narcotic, and if used in herbal medicine today, is used externally. An oil extracted from the leaves can be applied externally and used to reduce the pain of rheumatism.

Herb Bennet

Herb bennet or hemlock, *Conium maculatum*, is another poisonous herb. It is sedative and antispasmodic but is so effective in the latter role that its consumption can lead to paralysis of the motor centers. A further increase in consumption can lead to paralysis of the respiratory muscles and death by asphyxiation, as Socrates well knew. In smaller doses, it was used in the treatment of spastic disorders such as tetanus, epilepsy, cramps, paralysis agitans, and spasms of the larynx. When inhaled, it can help to relieve asthma, deep bronchial coughs, and whooping cough. However, it should not be taken without medical prescription and would almost certainly not be recommended or allowed today.

Hops

Humulus lupulus is anodyne, nervine, tonic and diuretic. A hops pillow, under your own, can help to improve sleep.

Horehound

See p.178.

Horseradish,

See p.247.

Hyssop

Hyssopus officinalis is astringent, carminative, emmenagogue, expectorant, stimulant, stomachic, and tonic, and is often used in combination with sage, which has similar properties. Gargle with it when you have a sore throat or catarrh. Swallow it to help your digestion; it will help to relieve flatulence, can support the liver in cases of jaundice, and can be used when there is mucus in the stool. It will help to relieve a cough associated with a cold or the flu.

Do not take it for prolonged periods; this herb is best used simply when the need arises. It can be used externally as a decoction on cuts, burns, and other wounds and for skin irritations.

Joe-Pye Weed

Eupartorium purpureum appears in gardening catalogs but is more commonly known in herbal manuals as gravelroot (See p.262).

Lady's Bedstraw

Our Lady's Bedstraw gets its name from its use by "ladies of rank," who could get the herb in sufficient quantity to stuff their mattresses with it. It has traditionally been used in cheese-making, particularly in the making of Cheshire cheese, as it has the ability to curdle milk. It is added with the rennet, and the yellow flowers add their color to the cheese. As a medicinal herb, *Galium verum* has been used in the treatment of urinary diseases and gravel.

Lady's Mantle

Alchemilla vulgaris is a strong astringent and styptic, very rich in tannin, and can be used to stop bleeding, both internally and externally. A decoction can be made from the root and used as a wash on wounds or on wet bandages to help dry up an open wound.

Lamb's Quarters

Chenopodium album is, like fat hen, a useful vegetable and can be used in place of spinach.

Larkspur, Wild

Delphinium consolida grows wild throughout the countryside. The seeds, made into a decoction, are used as a parasiticide and insecticide and as a wash to get rid of lice and nits in the hair. An infusion of the whole plant helps to settle digestion and particularly colic.

Lavender

Use the leaves and flowers of *Lavandula officinalis*. It is an antispasmodic, carminative, cholagogue, diuretic, sedative, stimulant, stomachic, and tonic.

It is generally used as the oil, and this is helpful in the treatment of headaches and migraines, fainting and dizzy spells. It can also be made into either an infusion or a decoction and used in the treatment of digestive problems, stomach and abdominal cramps, nausea and vomiting. The flowers can be added to a salad and help to relieve flatulence. The flowers and leaves, fresh or dried, can be made into a pillow using butter muslin. Placed under your own pillow, it can induce relaxation and sleep.

Lemon Balm

The leaves of *Melissa officinalis* are antispasmodic, calmative, carminative, diaphoretic, emmenagogue, and stomachic. For our purposes, this is useful for stomach problems and poor digestion and helps to relieve dyspepsia, flatulence, stomach and abdominal cramps, and colic. It is also helpful in the treatment of catarrhal problems and asthma.

Drink this herb if you have a headache or migraine or have trouble getting to sleep. You can also put it under your pillow. Externally the leaves can be used as a poultice for skin problems and insect bites.

This is an excellent herb to use when you want the flavor of lemon in a dish, but without the bitterness. The same is true of lemon grass. Make an infusion of either herb, and use this liquid as appropriate.

Lemon Grass

See p.248.

Licorice

See p.110.

Lobelia

See p.179.

Loosestrife

Lythrum salicaria, also known as purple willow herb or rainbow weed, is an astringent styptic useful in the treatment of diarrhea, including that associated with serious illnesses such as typhoid fever and dysentery. It can be used as an infusion, even by children and infants.

Lovage

Levisticum officinale grows robustly up to five or six feet tall, then dies down and retires into its root in the winter, only to emerge with the same exuberance in the spring. It is carminative, diuretic, emmenagogue, expectorant, stimulant, and stomachic. The leaves taste like aromatic celery and make an excellent addition to salads or to flavor cream cheeses.

Its main use is as a diuretic and thus will help cleansing via the kidneys and urine. In addition, it helps digestion and to eliminate catarrh.

It should not be used during pregnancy and can bring on menstruation.

Madder

Rubia tinctorum is not generally used medicinally but is said to be useful in the treatment of amenorrhea and liver problems such as jaundice.

Mallow, Musk

Malva moschata has properties similar to those of marsh mallow, though not as strong.

Marigold

See p.196.

Marjoram, Sweet

See p.248, 249.

Marsh Mallow

See p.197.

Meadowsweet

Spiraea ulmaris, also known as queen of the meadow and a common wild plant, is aromatic, astringent, diuretic, and a mild alterative. It is thus helpful as a blood cleanser and useful in the treatment of digestive problems, particularly diarrhea, in both children and adults. An infusion can be made from the flowers and leaves.

Milk Thistle

See p.128.

Mugwort

Artemisia vulgaris is a stimulant tonic, nervine, emmenagogue, diuretic, and diaphoretic. Its main use, often in combination with pennyroyal, is as an emmenagogue, and so it should not be used during a desired and established pregnancy.

Mullein, Great

See p.180.

Mustard

See p.249.

Nasturtium

See p.147.

Nettle

See p.186.

Oregano

See p.249.

Pansy

It may seem unkind to eat the common pansy that graces so many flower beds, but *Viola tricolor* is anodyne, demulcent, diaphoretic, diuretic, expectorant, laxative, and vulnerary and so has many benefits to offer a Detox Regime. Use the flowers and leaves.

As an anodyne, it helps to relieve pain. As a demulcent and diuretic it helps with urinary problems and fluid retention. It has also helped children with problems of bed-wetting. It will help to relieve constipation and has been used in the treatment of jaundice. As a demulcent and expectorant, it helps to relieve catarrhal congestion.

Parsley

See p.250.

Pennyroyal

Hedeoma pulegioides is carminative, diaphoretic, emmenagogue, and sedative. It will help to relieve flatulence and has been used to encourage and relieve a fever. It should not be used during pregnancy, as it is among the stronger herbs that can bring on menstruation.

Peppermint

See p.251.

Periwinkle

There are two periwinkles, *Vinca major* and *Vinca minor*, and they are both astringent and tonic and are used to stop bleeding. Culpeper tells us it "stays bleeding at the mouth and nose, if it be chewed." It can also help to relieve heavy menstrual bleeding. The fresh herb can be readily used as a tea.

Plantain

Plantago major is deobstruent, diuretic, refrigerant, and a mild astringent. The leaves have been applied externally to the skin in cases of inflammation, and ulcers.

Pleurisy Root

See p.155.

Poke Root

See p.160.

Red Clover

See p.188.

Rock Rose

Also known as frostwort, its Latin name is *Helianthemum canadense*. It is antiscrofulous, astringent, alterative, and tonic. In past centuries and when syphilis was more common, it was used to treat secondary symptoms. It is still useful in the treatment of diarrhea and, as a wash, of ulcers and other scrofulous skin conditions.

Rosemary

See p.253.

Rue

Ruta graveolens, also known by the delightful name of Herb of Grace, is antispasmodic, anthelmintic, carminative, emmenagogue, stimulant, and stomachic. In large doses, it is emetic. Its main use is in the treatment of rheumatism and gout. As an antispasmodic, it is useful in the treatment of croupy coughs; and as an antispasmodic, it is useful in conditions of flatulence and intestinal colic. An infusion, sprinkled around the house or on affected animals, helps to repel fleas.

Rupturewort

Herniaria glabra is an effective diuretic and can be used for the treatment of edema or fluid retention, whether it is caused by kidney or heart problems.

Safflower

The flowers of *Carthamus tinctorius* are diaphoretic, diuretic, and laxative. An infusion will help to bring a fever gently to resolution and is particularly useful in such childhood complaints as chickenpox, measles, and other fevers. The infusion can also be drunk to increase perspiration and reduce a fever in influenza and feverish colds.

Sage

See p.254.

Santolini

Santolina chamaecyparissus, also known as lavender cotton, although it is not a true lavender, is a stimulant and vermifuge, especially useful for children. The dried plant, when spread among clothes and linens, helps to repel moths.

Scabious

Scabiosa success, also known as devil's bit, has a stunted, squared-off root. Legend has it that the devil found it in paradise, realized how beneficial it was, and so bit off part of the root as he tried, but failed, to make it a less useful herb. It is diaphoretic, demulcent, and febrifuge. The leaves can be made into a tea and used in the treatment of coughs, fevers, and internal inflammations. It can also be used as a wash for external cuts.

Scurvy Grass

Cochlearia officinalis grows readily in cool climates, such as occurs in northern Scotland as well as further south. The name comes from its use on ships' voyages to prevent scurvy. It follows that it is rich in vitamin C and bioflavonoids. It is stimulant, aperient, diuretic, and antiscorbutic. An infusion of the fleshy leaves should be made allowing ½ cup to 2 cups of water and drunk several times a day, in small quantities.

Skullcap

There are many different types of skullcap, but two of them, *Scutellaria galericulata* and *Scutellaria minor,* are commonly found growing wild in Britain. Skullcap is a strong tonic, nervine and antispasmodic and a mild astringent. It is most commonly used as a calming herb in the treatment of stress, particularly mental and nervous stress, tension, anxiety, insomnia, nervous and tension headaches and neuralgia. It relaxes the muscles and is used in the treatment of a number of convulsive disorders.

Soapwort

Saponaria officinalis is cholagogue, diuretic, expectorant and purgative. By stimulating the flow of bile, it can help in cases of congested liver and gall function and in constipation. As a diuretic, it can promote cleansing via the urine; and as an expectorant, it can promote the secretion of excess mucus and the treatment of respiratory congestion.

- The root of the plant should be used. Dry it, chop finely, and simmer one to two tablespoons per cup of water. Take one tablespoon of this three times a day.

Sorrel

The leaves of *Rumex acetosa* make an excellent addition to salads. They are refrigerant and diuretic, and the infusion makes a cooling drink when you have a temperature.

SORREL SOUP

Follow the recipe for Chervil Soup (p.241), replacing the chervil leaves with a large bunch of sorrel.

Spearmint

Spearmint, or *Mentha viridis*, is generally used in cooking. It has properties similar to, though weaker than, those of peppermint, being stimulant — carminative, and antispasmodic. As such, it aids the digestive system when incorporated into foods.

Speedwell

Veronica officinalis is commonly found growing wild in hedge-rows and on moors. It is diaphoretic, alterative, diuretic, expectorant, and tonic. It has been used extensively in the treatment of coughs and catarrh, and so has a clear place in a Detox program if the lungs and upper respiratory system need to be cleared out.

Strawberry, Wild

The name *strawberry* has nothing to do with the habit of putting straw under the berries to protect them. The name is older and comes from "to strew," and the plant's habit of throwing out suckers and spreading itself over the ground with great energy.

Fragaria vesca, unlike its fleshier fruit variety, is readily found growing wild. The berries, though smaller, have a strong and fragrant flavor. Medicinally it is a laxative, diuretic, and astringent, and so useful in a Detox program. The astringent action is useful in the treatment of diarrhea, and the laxative action in the treatment of constipation. This is a common action of herbal remedies, to treat the two extremes and so to balance the system. It is also useful in the treatment of rheumatism and gout. The fruit can be eaten, and the leaves, or both, made into an infusion.

The fresh juice of the fruit can be rubbed on the teeth (and brushed off using bicarbonate of soda five minutes later) to reduce discoloration, or rubbed on the skin for the same reason. A pulp made from the fruit and allowed to sit on the skin for half an hour can help in cases of sunburn.

St John's Wort

Hypericum perforatum is aromatic, astringent, expectorant, and nervine, the latter being the use for which it is currently best known. It is useful in the treatment of lung problems and in cases where there is restricted urine production and output. In the digestive system, it is used in the treatment of diarrhea, dysentery, and worms. It is also used for mental problems including the treatment of nervous depression.

- A quarter cup of the herb should be infused in two cups of water and one to two tablespoons of this liquid taken two or three times a day.

Summer Savory

Satureja hortensis is astringent, carminative, expectorant, stimulant, and stomachic. It is most commonly used for digestive problems, helping in cases of nausea, stomach and intestinal cramps, and lack of appetite. Its astringent action helps in cases of diarrhea and it can be used as a gargle for throat problems.

Sunflower

Gardeners will think of the wonderful yellow blooms on a plant that grows several feet tall. Those interested in healthy snacks will think of the seeds as being highly nutritious. *Helianthus annuus* also has other uses.

Medicinally, the seeds are diuretic and expectorant. A decoction of the crushed seeds is useful in the treatment of bronchial problems, as is an infusion made from the flowers and leaves.

Sweet Cicely

Myrrhis odorata is aromatic, stomachic, carminative, and expectorant. The roots are antiseptic. A decoction of the root makes a good gargle for coughs and irritable throats; swallow afterwards and it will ease indigestion. The root can also be eaten.

LOW-SUGAR RHUBARB

The leaves of sweet cicely are particularly useful as a sugar substitute. It is not that they are sweet in themselves, but they do reduce the bitterness of many fruits. I have heard it said that they do this by blocking the taste buds that detect the sourness and acidity. Be that as it may, I grow it next to the rhubarb plants, and that reminds me to put a generous bunch of the leaves into the pot when I am steaming the rhubarb. When you do this, you can reduce the amount of sugar to half or less.

You need 6 large or 12 small stems of rhubarb. Clean them, chop, and place in a saucepan with just a teaspoon or two of water to moisten the base. You do not need more, provided you apply very low heat, as the juice soon comes out of the rhubarb itself and you will have plenty of liquid. Add several generous sprigs of sweet cicely, keeping the herb intact so you can remove it after cooking, and one teaspoon of honey. Cook slowly until the fruit has softened, and adjust the sweetness to taste. For something different, you can replace the few teaspoons of water that you use initially with a splash of port — delicious.

LEMON DESSERTS WITHOUT SUGAR

You can, of course, do the same thing with other fruits. Next time you add lemon juice to a recipe, see if you can't also add an infusion or decoction of sweet cicely. It will depend, of course, on whether or not any other liquid is used.

Tansy

See p.119.

Tarragon

See p.254.

Thyme

See p.89.

Tormentil

Potentilla tormentilla, or shepherds' knot, is a perennial and grows wild in damp and marshy places. The rhizome is astringent, useful in the treatment of diarrhea and in other conditions where there is a discharge. A decoction can be used as a gargle for treatment for a sore, tired, or ulcerated throat. A stronger decoction is helpful, when locally applied, in the treatment of hemorrhoids and to reduce the bleeding of cuts and other wounds.

- To make the decoction for internal use, allow 1 teaspoon per cup and simmer for 10 minutes. For external use, allow a cup to a cup, simmer for 15 minutes, and strain.

Valerian

See p.254.

Vervain, Blue

See p.135.

Winter Savory

Satureja montana is a perennial shrub. It is more woody than summer savory, but some say it has similar medicinal properties. According to other authorities, the leaves have little medicinal use, but mixed with breadcrumbs, it has been used "to breade their meate, be it fish or flesh, to give it a quicker relish."

Woodruff, Sweet

Asperula odorata is an antispasmodic, calmative, cardiac, diaphoretic, and diuretic. It has been used to reduce the pain of headaches, migraines, and neuralgia. As a calmative, it can be used to treat stress and nervous tension, also for insomnia and restless sleep. It has been used in the treatment of jaundice and is helpful if there is a tendency toward bladder stones or gravel.

• Make an infusion allowing one teaspoon of the dried herb per cup for the treatment of stomach pain or for an irregular heartbeat. You should not exceed this dose.

Wormwood

See p.94.

Yarrow

See p.171.

✦✦✦ ✦✦✦

+ +

Internet Sources

At the time of going to press, the site **www.herbalmedicine.com** leads to several sub-groups under the headings of "medicinal herb," "herbal remedy" and "herbal medicine." The total is such that the list is too long to list here. However, a search for yourself will almost certainly lead you to whatever herb you want.

✦ ✦

Glossary

adipose tissue	fatty tissues in the body
alkali	the opposite of an acid
allergen	a substance to which a person is allergic
alterative	an herb or other substance that helps to remove toxins from the blood stream, commonly referred to as a "blood cleanser"
amenorrhoea	the absence of menstrual periods during a woman's reproductive years
antibodies	substances in the blood which destroy antigens
antigen	a substance, usually a protein, that is foreign to the body, and that causes the formation of antibodies within the body
anthelmintic	an herb or other substance that acts against intestinal parasites
astringent	an herb or other substance that tightens tissues by acting on the tissue proteins
atheroma	a degenerative change within the walls of the arteries
bioflavonoids	a group of compounds found in plants, usually associated with and acting with vitamin C

bitter	an herb or other substance that stimulates digestion, particularly the flow of stomach acid
bolus	a lump of food, prepared for swallowing by the action of saliva
Candida albicans	an organism which can exist in mold or fungi form and is responsible for the symptoms associated with candidiasis
carcinogen	a substance that can cause cells to become cancerous
carminative	an herb or other substance that reduces flatulence
chelating agent	a type of compound that combines with ions, usually metal ions
colitis	inflammation of the colon
demulcent	an herb or other substance that contains mucilaginous components and is soothing and protective
diverticuli	pouches that can form in the walls of the colon
diverticulitis	inflammed diverticuli
DHEA	Dehydroepiandrosterone
dyspepsia	indigestion felt in the chest or upper abdomen, usually involving heartburn, nausea, and pain
enzyme	a biological catalyst synthesis of which is controlled by the genetic code in the cells
hydroxylate	to add hydroxyl groups, part of the water molecule

hypocholesterolemic | low level of cholesterol in the blood

hypolipidemic | a low level of lipids or fats in the blood

laxative | an herb or other substance that stimulates bowel action; a strong laxative can cause diarrhea

mucilage | viscous substance produced by plants

pathogen | a harmful organism

phagocytosis | the action a cell performs when it encloses and engulfs an external substance or microorganism

proanthocyanidins | colorless compounds, related to bioflavonoids, that can convert towards red; physiologically active, commonly associated with vitamin C

prophylactic | a substance or action that prevents an otherwise possible or likely outcome

prostatitis | inflammation of the prostate gland

psoriasis | a skin disease characterized by raised red patches and scaly flakes of dead skin

purgative | a very strong laxative that causes significant evacuation of the colon

putrefaction | the progressive decomposition of organic matter, usually proteins and usually in the absence of oxygen

rhizome | prostrate root-like stem, sends out roots

sepsis | infection or poisoning caused by the growth of microorganisms

sialogogue

an herb or other substance that stimulates the flow of saliva

tincture

the solution obtained when the active
ingredients of an herb are extracted into
a strong alcohol solution

vasodilator

an herb or other substance that causes
the veins and capillaries to dilate

✦✦✦   ✦✦✦

✦ ✦
Useful Tables

Table i gives you a list of the herbs that have been mentioned in this book and indicates their actions. Use this table to find, for instance, a list of the carminative herbs or alterative herbs. You can use this table to find which herb covers several different actions that are relevant to you.

You might want an herb that is a carminative and nervine. By looking along the rows, you could pick out centaury and peppermint as your two options.

Table ii will help you find you way around this book. Because herbs act on more than one part of the body, you will not always find their full description in the section in which you are interested. Use this chart to find descriptions of the herbs that interest you.

MAIN indicates the section or chapter in which the main description of the herb is given.

OTHER indicates the sections or chapters in which further information is given on the herb.

Table iii The nutrient content of herbs. Unfortunately, there is relatively little information available as to the nutrient content of herbs. Some is given in this table. However, gaps in the table do not necessarily indicate a lack of the nutrient; it may be lack of information. Most plants, and particularly the leaves, are rich sources of many vitamins, the ones included in the table and vitamins B5, B6, folic acid, and vitamin K. Many herbs also contain trace minerals in addition to the major minerals noted. However, given the quantity of an herb that is usually consumed, the amounts provided would be small. Nonetheless, the generous addition of herbs and leaves to your diet is likely to make a significant contribution to the overall nutrient value of your diet. *, **, and *** indicate increasing amounts, x indicating significant amounts.

Sources: John Lust, *The Herb Book, A Nutri Book* and US Department of Agriculture, Bulletin 8.

✦✦✦   ✦✦✦

Table i Part A

Herb	Alterative	Analgesic	Anodyne	Anthelmintic	Antiasthmatic	Antibilious	Anticatarrhal	Anticoagulant	Antiemetic	Antifungal	Antihaemorrhagic	Antihistamine	Anti-inflammatory	Antilithic	Antimicrobial	Antineoplastic	Antioxidant	Antirheumatic	Antiscorbutic	Antiseptic	Antispasmodic	Antitussive	Antiviral	Aperient	Aromatic	Astringent	Bitter
Agrimony																											
Ajowan																											
Alexanders																											
Alfalfa																											
Alkanet																											
Allspice																									X		
Aloe																											
Angelica																					X						
Aniseed																					X				X		
Arnica																											
Balm of Gilead																											
Balmony									X																		
Barberry																											
Basil																					X						
Bay																									X	X	
Bearberry																				X						X	
Bergamot																											
Bistort																											
Black Root																					X						
Blessed Thistle																											
Blue Flag	X												X														
Bogbean																		X									X
Bog Myrtle																											
Boldo																											
Boneset																					X		X				
Borage													X														
Broom																											
Buchu																				X							
Buckwheat																											
Burdock	X																										X
Campion																											
Caper																											
Caraway																					X				X	X	
Cardamon																									X		
Cascara																											X
Catnip																					X					X	
Cat's Claw													X		X	X					X		X				
Cayenne		X							X									X		X							X
Celery																		X									
Centaury																									X		X
Chamomile		X											X							X	X						
Chervil																											
Chicory																											
Chickweed																		X									
Chives																									X		
Cinnamon																									X	X	

Cardiac tonic	Carminative	Cathartic	Cholagogue	Circulatory stimulant	Demulcent	Diaphoretic	Digestive stimulant	Diuretic	Emetic	Emmenagogue	Emollient	Expectorant	Febrifuge	Galactogue	Gastric stimulant	Hepatic	Hypnotic	Hypotensive	Laxative	Nervine	Oxytocic	Parasiticide	Pectoral	Purgative	Respiratory stimulant	Rubefacient	Sedative	Sialogogue	Stimulant	Stomach tonic	Tonic	Vermifuge	Vulnerary
X						X																											
	X		X						X	X																						X	X
X				X		X						X																					
X												X										X											
		X														X													X				
							X																								X		
X							X																							X			
			X				X																										
	X	X			X																												
			X					X											X														
			X					X																									
			X					X							X										X								
					X																										X		
					X						X		X																		X		
							X																										
							X																										
X									X	X	X																						
X																												X					
																								X							X		
X					X																												
X																									X						X		
	X																									X	X	X		X			
X						X																				X							
														X					X														
X																																	X
								X	X			X																					
										X																							X
						X																											
X																														X			

Table i — Part B

Herb	Alterative	Analgesic	Anodyne	Anthelmintic	Antiasthmatic	Antibilious	Anticatarrhal	Anticoagulant	Antiemetic	Antifungal	Antihaemorrhagic	Antihistamine	Anti-inflammatory	Antilithic	Antimicrobial	Antineoplastic	Antioxidant	Antirheumatic	Antiscorbutic	Antiseptic	Antispasmodic	Antitussive	Antiviral	Aperient	Aromatic	Astringent	Bitter
Cleavers	X										X				X											X	
Cloves																									X		
Coltsfoot							X															X					
Columbine																											
Comfrey																										X	
Coreopsis																											
Coriander (Cilantro)																									X		
Cornsilk																											
Couch Grass															X												
Cranesbill											X		X													X	
Cucumber																											
Cumin																					X						
Daisy																											
Dandelion																		X									
Dill																					X				X		
Dog Rose																											
Echinacea	X														X												
Elder							X																				
Elecampane															X							X					
Epazote																											
Eucalyptus																											
Evening Primrose																											
Fennel																					X				X		
Fenugreek																											
Feverfew																											
Figwort	X																										
Flax																											
Fleabane																											
Fringe Tree	X					X																					
Fuller's Teasel																											
Fumitory	X																										
Garlic																				X	X		X				
Gentian																											X
Germander																											
Ginger		X							X		X	X															
Gipsy Wort																											
Goat's Rue																											
Golden Seal							X																			X	X
Good King Henry																											
Greater Celandine			X																		X						
Greater Knapweed																											
Greenwood Dyer's																											
Grindelia																					X						
Heartsease																											
Heather, Ling																											
Hemp																											

Cardiac tonic	Carminative	Cathartic	Cholagogue	Circulatory stimulant	Demulcent	Diaphoretic	Digestive stimulant	Diuretic	Emetic	Emmenagogue	Emollient	Expectorant	Febrifuge	Galactogue	Gastric stimulant	Hepatic	Hypnotic	Hypotensive	Laxative	Nervine	Oxytocic	Parasiticide	Pectoral	Purgative	Respiratory stimulant	Rubefacient	Sedative	Sialogogue	Stimulant	Stomach tonic	Tonic	Vermifuge	Vulnerary
								X																							X		
X																													X				
			X					X				X																					
			X									X																					X
X																																	
			X					X																					X				
			X					X																									
																																	X
			X					X																									X
X																													X				
	X							X								X			X										X				
X													X																				
					X			X	X			X							X					X									
					X							X														X							
X								X	X																	X			X				
						X		X	X																					X			
X								X																X									
		X						X								X			X											X			
								X											X														
					X		X									X																	
					X									X														X					
X				X	X																					X			X				
																	X	X													X		
		X						X																X									
												X							X														

Table i — Part C

Herb	Alterative	Analgesic	Anodyne	Anthelmintic	Antiasthmatic	Antibilious	Anticatarrhal	Anticoagulant	Antiemetic	Antifungal	Antihaemorrhagic	Antihistamine	Anti-inflammatory	Antilithic	Antimicrobial	Antineoplastic	Antioxidant	Antirheumatic	Antiscorbutic	Antiseptic	Antispasmodic	Antitussive	Antiviral	Aperient	Aromatic	Astringent	Bitter
Henbane																											
Herb Bennet																											
Hollyhock, Black																											
Hops																											
Horehound																					X						X
Horseradish																											
Horsetail																										X	
Hound's Tongue																											
Hyssop																					X						
Indigo																											
Iris Flag																											
Irish Moss																											
Jacob's Ladder																											
Joe-Pye Weed, Gravelroot																											
Juniper																		X			X						
Knitbone																											
Lady's Bedstraw																											
Lady's Mantle																											
Larkspur																											
Lavender																											
Lemon Balm																					X						
Lemon Grass																											
Lesser Calamint																											
Liquorice													X								X						
Lobelia					X																X						
Lungwort																										X	
Madder																											
Mallow, Common																											
Mallow, Musk																											
Marigold										X			X													X	
Marjoram																											
Marsh Mallow																											
Meadowsweet																											
Milk Thistle																											
Mole Plant																											
Motherwort																											
Mountain Grape	X						X			X																	
Motherwort																											
Mullein																											
Mustard																											
Myrrh							X								X											X	
Myrtle																											
Nasturtium															X												
Nigella																											
Nettles																										X	
Nutmeg																									X		

Cardiac tonic	Carminative	Cathartic	Cholagogue	Circulatory stimulant	Demulcent	Diaphoretic	Digestive stimulant	Diuretic	Emetic	Emmenagogue	Emollient	Expectorant	Febrifuge	Galactogue	Gastric stimulant	Hepatic	Hypnotic	Hypotensive	Laxative	Nervine	Oxytocic	Parasiticide	Pectoral	Purgative	Respiratory stimulant	Rubefacient	Sedative	Sialogogue	Stimulant	Stomach tonic	Tonic	Vermifuge	Vulnerary
												X																					X
X								X										X									X			X			
								X																									X
X							X					X														X							
					X							X																					
X								X																									
X								X											X														
																														X			
					X	X						X							X														
							X		X			X												X									
					X							X																					X
		X							X																								X
					X				X			X	X																				X
		X	X												X																		
					X													X													X		
		X						X				X																X					X
								X	X																	X			X				
X												X																					X
								X																							X		
X																													X				

Table i Part D

Herb	Alterative	Analgesic	Anodyne	Anthelmintic	Antiasthmatic	Antibilious	Anticatarrhal	Anticoagulant	Antiemetic	Antifungal	Antihaemorrhagic	Antihistamine	Anti-inflammatory	Antilithic	Antimicrobial	Antineoplastic	Antioxidant	Antirheumatic	Antiscorbutic	Antiseptic	Antispasmodic	Antitussive	Antiviral	Aperient	Aromatic	Astringent	Bitter
Oreganum																				X							
Oxeye Daisy																											
Pansy																											
Parsley																											
Pasque Flower		X													X					X							
Pennyroyal																											
Peppermint		X							X											X	X		X				
Periwinkle																											
Plantain																											
Pleurisy Root																											
Poke Root							X											X									
Pumpkin seeds				X																							
Purple Loosestrife																											
Purslane																											
Pyrethrum																											
Quassia				X																							X
Rampion																											
Red Clover	X															X				X							
Rock Rose																											
Rosehip																							X		X		
Roselle																											
Rosemary																				X	X		X				
Rhubarb Root																										X	X
Rucola																											
Rue																											
Rupturewort																											
Safflower																											
Saffron			X																		X						
Sage																				X					X		
Santolini																											
Sarsparilla	X																X										
Sassafras	X																										
Scabious																											
Scurvy Grass																											
Seaholly, Field																											
Seaholly																											
Self Heal																										X	
Senna																											
Skullcap																											
Slippery Elm																										X	
Soapwort																											
Sorrel																											
Spearmint																											
Strawberry Sticks																											
Spinach																											
Strawberry, Wild																											
St. John's Wort																											

Cardiac tonic	Carminative	Cathartic	Cholagogue	Circulatory stimulant	Demulcent	Diaphoretic	Digestive stimulant	Diuretic	Emetic	Emmenagogue	Emollient	Expectorant	Febrifuge	Galactogue	Gastric stimulant	Hepatic	Hypnotic	Hypotensive	Laxative	Nervine	Oxytocic	Parasiticide	Pectoral	Purgative	Respiratory stimulant	Rubefacient	Sedative	Sialogogue	Stimulant	Stomach tonic	Tonic	Vermifuge	Vulnerary
						X				X		X													X				X				
X								X		X		X																					
																												X					
X						X				X																			X				
X						X												X															
									X															X					X				
																												X					
										X																							
						X																											
X																				X				X									
																		X					X										
									X			X																X					
X																																	
					X			X																									
X					X			X																									
																															X		X
	X																																
		X								X																							
						X		X				X							X														

Table i Part E

Herb	Alterative	Analgesic	Anodyne	Anthelmintic	Antiasthmatic	Antibilious	Anticatarrhal	Anticoagulant	Antiemetic	Antifungal	Antihaemorrhagic	Antihistamine	Anti-inflammatory	Antilithic	Antimicrobial	Antineoplastic	Antioxidant	Antirheumatic	Antiscorbutic	Antiseptic	Antispasmodic	Antitussive	Antiviral	Aperient	Aromatic	Astringent	Bitter
Sunflower																											
Sweet Cicely																											
Tansy				X																							X
Tarragon																											
Tea Tree																											
Thistle, Scottish																											
Thorn Apple																											
Toadflax, common																											
Tormentil																											
Traveller's Joy																											
Thuja	X																									X	
Thyme				X						X					X			X			X					X	
Turmeric																	X								X		
Valerian																					X						
Vanilla Grass																											
Vervain																					X						
Viper's Bugloss																											
Vitex Neguno																											
Wahoo																											
Weld, Dyers Rocket																											
Wild Indigo							X								X												
Wild Yam													X					X			X						
Winter Savoury																											
Witch Hazel																										X	
Woodruff, Sweet																											
Wormwood				X									X														X
Woundwort																				X	X					X	
Yarrow																					X						
Yellow Dock	X																										
TOP TEN																											
Gentian																											X
Milk Thistle																											
Rhubarb Root																										X	X
Cat's Claw													X				X				X		X				
Poke Root							X											X									
Buchu																				X							
Coltsfoot							X															X					
Red Clover	X															X					X						
Golden Seal							X																			X	X
Ginseng																											
Schizandra																X	X										
Blackberry leaves																										X	
Pansy			X																								
Primrose			X																								

Cardiac tonic	Carminative	Cathartic	Cholagogue	Circulatory stimulant	Demulcent	Diaphoretic	Digestive stimulant	Diuretic	Emetic	Emmenagogue	Emollient	Expectorant	Febrifuge	Galactogue	Gastric stimulant	Hepatic	Hypnotic	Hypotensive	Laxative	Nervine	Oxytocic	Parasiticide	Pectoral	Purgative	Respiratory stimulant	Rubefacient	Sedative	Sialogogue	Stimulant	Stomach tonic	Tonic	Vermifuge	Vulnerary
	X									X																						X	
								X																						X			
								X				X																					
X												X																					
																												X					
X																		X									X						
							X						X		X				X								X						
			X	X				X											X														
										X																							
		X																															
X																																	
																																	X
							X	X										X															
		X																						X									
		X													X													X					
		X		X									X																				
																		X			X												
X																					X										X		
								X													X								X				
							X																										
			X				X				X																						
							X																										
																		X		X											X		
																													X		X		
										X																					X		
			X	X				X		X									X														X
								X		X																							

Table ii Part A Herb	Colon	Immune	Kidneys	Liver	Lungs	Lymph	Mouth	Parasites	Skin	Stomach	Culinary
Allspice											MAIN
Aloe									other	MAIN	
Angelica		MAIN									other
Aniseed											MAIN
Balmony				MAIN							
Barberry				MAIN						other	
Basil									other		MAIN
Bay											MAIN
Bearberry			MAIN								
Birch			MAIN								
Black Root				MAIN							
Black Walnut								MAIN			
Blue Flag				MAIN					other		
Bogbean	MAIN										
Boldo			other	MAIN							
Boneset		MAIN									
Borage											
Buchu		MAIN									
Burdock									MAIN		
Butternut								MAIN			
Cardamon											MAIN
Carraway											MAIN
Cascara	MAIN										
Catnip		MAIN									
Cat's Claw		MAIN									
Cayenne		other					MAIN				
Celery			MAIN								other
Centaury						other				MAIN	
Chamomile											MAIN
Chervil											MAIN
Chickweed									MAIN		
Chives											MAIN
Cinnamon											MAIN
Cleavers			other			MAIN			other		
Cloves											MAIN
Coltsfoot					MAIN						
Comfrey					MAIN				other		
Coriander (Cilantro)											MAIN
Cornsilk											MAIN
Couch grass			MAIN								
Cucumber											MAIN
Cumin											MAIN
Daisy					MAIN						
Dandelion	other		other	MAIN							
Dill											MAIN

Table ii Part B Herb	Colon	Immune	Kidneys	Liver	Lungs	Lymph	Mouth	Parasites	Skin	Stomach	Culinary
Echinacaea		MAIN							other		
Elder	other	MAIN									
Elecampane					MAIN						
Eucalyptus		other							MAIN		
Fennel											MAIN
Fenugreek											MAIN
Figwort									MAIN		
Fringe Tree	other			MAIN							
Fumitory									MAIN		
Garlic		MAIN						other			other
Gentian							other			MAIN	
Ginger		other					MAIN	other			other
Golden Seal	other			other		MAIN		other	other	MAIN	
Greater Celandine				MAIN							
Grindelia					MAIN						
Horehound					MAIN			other			
Horseradish											MAIN
Horsetail									MAIN		
Hyssop		MAIN									
Irish Moss									MAIN		
Juniper			MAIN								other
Lemon Grass											MAIN
Linseeds	MAIN				other				other		other
Licorice	MAIN	other					other				other
Lobelia					MAIN						
Lungwort					MAIN						
Marigold								other	MAIN		
Marjoram											MAIN
Marsh Mallow									MAIN		
Milk Thistle	other			MAIN							
Mullein					MAIN						
Mustard											MAIN
Myrrh		MAIN									
Nasturtium		MAIN									
Nettle									MAIN		
Nutmeg											MAIN
Olive									MAIN		other
Oreganum											MAIN
Parsley											MAIN
Pau D'Arco								MAIN			
Peppermint		other								MAIN	other
Pleurisy Root		other			other						
Poke Root					other	MAIN			other		
Psyllium Hulls	MAIN										
Pumpkin								MAIN			other

Table ii Part C Herb	Colon	Immune	Kidneys	Liver	Lungs	Lymph	Mouth	Parasites	Skin	Stomach	Culinary
Quassia								other			other
Red Clover					other				SKIN		
Rhubarb Root	MAIN										
Rosehip											MAIN
Rosemary											MAIN
Saffron											MAIN
Sage											MAIN
Sarsparilla									MAIN		
Sassafras									MAIN		
Senna	MAIN										
Slippery Elm	MAIN								MAIN		
Spearmint											MAIN
Tansy								MAIN			
Tarragon											MAIN
Thuja					MAIN				other		
Thyme		other					MAIN	other	other		other
Turmeric											MAIN
Valerian											MAIN
Vervain				MAIN							
Wahoo	other			MAIN							
Wild Indigo						MAIN					
Wild Yam	MAIN										
Witch Hazel									MAIN		
Wormwood									other	MAIN	
Yarrow		other	MAIN								
Yellow Dock				MAIN					other		

Table iii Part A — Herb	Carotene	Vitamin B1	Vitamin B2	Vitamin B3	Vitamin B5	Vitamin B6	Folic acid	Vitamin C	Vitamin E	Vitamin K	Calcium	Iron	Magnesium	Potassium
Alfalfa	X		X	X	X		X	X			X		X	X
Boneset								**						
Borage	X			X				X			X	X	X	*
Burdock Root				X				X			X		X	X
Calendula	*													
Cascara												*		
Catnip								**						
Cayenne	X			X				*					*	
Centaury, American														*
Chamomile														*
Chickweed								*						
Chives		X	X	X	X	X		X			X		X	X
Cleavers												*		
Coltsfoot								*				*		*
Comfrey														*
Coriander	X		X	X				X			X	X	X	X
Cowslip, flowers	*													
Dandelion, leaves	***	**	*	*					**		**	**	*	**
Elderberries	**							*			**			**
Elecampane, flowers	*													
Fennel														*
Fenugreek, seed				*										
Garlic	*	X	X	X			X	*				X		X
Ginger				X	X	X		X					X	X
Horseradish								*						X
Knotgrass								*						
Lamb's Quarters	***	*	*	*				**			**		X	
Milfoil														*
Mulein														*
Mustard Greens	*	*	*	*	X			**			**	**		**
Nettle	**							**			*			*
Parsley	**		X	**	X	X	X	***			**	**	*	**
Peppermint												*	*	*
Plantain, lance-leaf														*
Pokeweed, young shoots	**			X				**			**			
Primrose, leaves													*	*
Purslane	X		X	X				X			**	**	X	X
Sage				*										
Savoury														*
Shave Grass												*		
Shepherd's Purse												*		*
Sorrel								*				*		
Spearmint	**							**						
Watercress	*	**	*	*	X	X		**			**		*	**
Wild Strawberry, leaves								***						

Table iii Part B Herb	Carotene	Vitamin B1	Vitamin B2	Vitamin B3	Vitamin B5	Vitamin B6	Folic acid	Vitamin C	Vitamin E	Vitamin K	Calcium	Iron	Magnesium	Potassium
Winter Cress	**							**						
Wormwood								*						
Yellow Dock	***		X	X				**			**		X	X

✦ ✦

Index

Please note: the location of the dosage information for a particular herb is indicated in bold type.

✛ ✛ ✛   ✛ ✛ ✛

✦ ✦ ✦

We hope you enjoyed this Hay House book.
If you would like to receive a free catalog featuring
additional Hay House books and products, or if you
would like information about the Hay Foundation,
please contact:

Hay House, Inc.
P.O. Box 5100
Carlsbad, CA 92018-5100

(760) 431-7695 or **(800) 654-5126**
(760) 431-6948 (fax) or **(800) 650-5115 (fax)**
www.hayhouse.com

✦ ✦ ✦

Published and distributed in Australia by:
Hay House Australia Pty Ltd, P.O. Box 515,
Brighton-Le-Sands, NSW 2216 • *phone:* 1800 023 516
e-mail: info@hayhouse.com.au

Distributed in Canada by:
Raincoast, 9050 Shaughnessy St.,
Vancouver, B.C., Canada V6P 6E5

✦ ✦ ✦